*S*it quietly with closed eyes. Imagine that you are reaching up,

grabbing a pleasant memory from your childhood—much like

taking hold of the string of a helium-filled balloon. Whatever the

memory, allow the details to drift; hold only to the pleasant remem-

brance of that memory's spirit. Perhaps you feel a warmth,

a sense of security, a calm assuredness that all is right.

Whatever that feeling, bathe yourself in it now.

Let the quality of simplicity surround you like a springtime breeze

in mid-afternoon. Simple, carefree, trusting—these are the qualities

washing from your thoughts all stress, over-concern, and overwhelm.

Now relax even more deeply. Visualize yourself at the foot

of a small forested hill. The sun-cloaked pine branches beckon you

forward. A few yards ahead, a young fawn dashes onto the footpath,

startling both of you. She freezes; you crouch down slowly.

She responds to your inner voice that says, "Don't be afraid. I'm

as curious as you." Her tiny ears draw back in timid wonder. Too young

to know fear and sensing your gentleness, she steps forward and sniffs

your outstretched palm. As she does so, you look into her eyes

so new to this world. You see in them the joy of new life and

the simple magic of childhood. Embrace the memory of the

fawn's eyes, again like taking hold of a balloon.

Remember that you too cradle a child inside.

The
ESSENTIAL

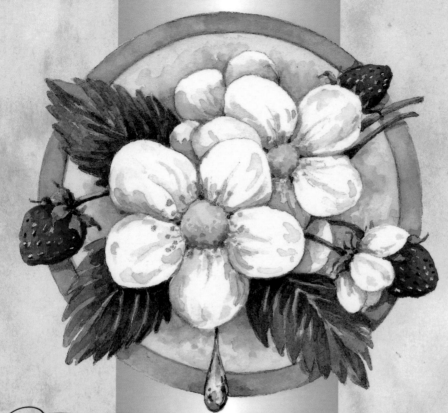

Flower Essence
HANDBOOK

Lila Devi

featuring

THE ORIGINAL
Spirit-in-Nature Essences™

REVISED EDITION

Ananda Blue Lotus
Meditation Temple,
Bothell

THE Essential Flower Essence Handbook

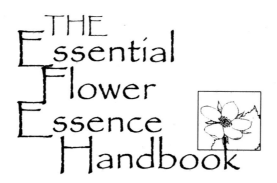

THE Essential Flower Essence Handbook

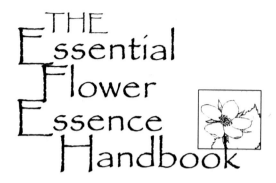

FOR
PERFECT
WELL-BEING

Lila Devi

Featuring

THE ORIGINAL
Spirit-in-Nature Essences™

Crystal Clarity Publishers
Nevada City, California

Crystal Clarity Publishers • Nevada City, CA 95959

First edition 1996. Second edition 1997. Third edition 1997. Fourth edition 2007
Printed in United States of America
Originally published in 1996 by Master's Flower Essences™

ISBN: 978-1-56589-081-7

Design: Jerianne Van Dijk and Kim Rogers • Typesetting: Kim Rogers
Back Cover photo: Barbara Bingham • Illustrations: Kaleigh Surber

The author of this book does not dispense medical advice or prescribe the use of any technique as a form of treatment for physical or medical problems without the advice of a physician, either directly or indirectly. The intent of the author is only to offer information of a general nature to help you in your quest for emotional and spiritual well-being. In the event you use any of the information in this book for yourself, which is your constitutional right, the author and the publisher assume no responsibility for your actions.

Library of Congress Cataloging-in-Publication Data
Devi, Lila
  The essential flower essence handbook for perfect well-being / Lila Devi — 4th ed.
     p. cm.
  Originally published: Nevada City, CA : Master's Flower Essences, 1996.
  Includes bibliographical references and index.
  ISBN 978-1-56589-081-7
  1. Flowers--Therapeutic use. I. Title.

  RX615.F55D48 2009
  615.8′515—dc22
                                        2009007313800.424.1055 or

530.478.7600
clarity@crystalclarity.com
www.crystalclarity.com

DEDICATION

To every flower that stills one's breath,

And every life lived fully till death.

To every friend, family and fawn,

And every dusk that hastens toward dawn.

To all of these, to all unseen,

To the humble flowers that we've always been.

To who we each are, to what we'll become—

Blossoms unfolding in noonday's glad sun.

DISCLAIMER

This book is a reference work not intended to treat, diagnose or prescribe. The information contained herein is in no way considered as a replacement for consultation with a duly licensed health-care professional.

ACKNOWLEDGEMENTS

With gratitude to all those who have so graciously provided their stories for this text; to J. Donald Walters, friend and guiding light; Cathy Parojinog, for her priceless editorial midwifery; Jon Caswell, for editing and encouragement; Sara Cryer, for the beauty of the logo and back cover text; Bhakti Rinzler, for her strawberry soup and other fine recipes (see the appendices); George Beinhorn, who always had a moment to inspire; with last-minute computer work, John Parkin; LeeAnn Brook for her depth of vision with the book cover and interior design; Rob Froelick, who has elevated typesetting to an art form; Kim Rogers, for the revised typesetting; Kaleigh Surber, for her sensitively rendered illustrations; to Merrily Beck, for taking charge in the office while I wrote this book; my wonderful parents; the many goats who herded my dreams; my dear friends in the hundreds whose smiles alone uplift; and ever to Paramhansa Yogananda.

CONTENTS

INTRODUCTION

In celebration of our 30-year anniversary in 2007, we have taken the new name of Spirit-in-Nature Essences, previously called Master's Flower Essences. This change has received an overwhelmingly positive response. Why the new name? It represents a new cycle, a new energy, and a more expansive description of what we're all about. These essences are about finding the Spirit in Nature—within Mother Nature, and within our own nature.

This is a book about becoming the master of your life. Self-mastery is more than a vague goal; it is an attainable state. How? In addition to healthy living, by keeping ourselves in a state of balance *through the wise use of flower essences.*

Flower essences stimulate our positive, spiritual qualities. They are prepared, simply, by extracting the life force from blossoms through the elements of sunlight and pure spring water. They introduce into our energy fields elevating vibrational examples of different ennobling qualities from the plant kingdom, such as dignity, kindness, and unconditional love.

Indeed, we cannot control the events that befall us; but we *can* control how we choose to respond to them. How will we spend the time allotted to us between the baby rattle and the death rattle? Perhaps you feel your boss has unjustly chastised you. Then your husband, himself overworked, greets your return home from a day at the office with short-tempered words. How will you react? Life's endless pitch of curve balls is designed, it seems, to throw us off center. Balance, harmony, and perfect well-being—these are the qualities to which we consciously aspire. The question is, how do we get there?

It may seem that flower essences are just a little too over-simplified for our complicated lives. How can something so subtle affect our consciousness so deeply? Through the vital force embodied in the essences, that very life-stuff of which we are made. If we were to try to revive a dead man with life-sustaining resources such as food, air, or water, nothing would happen. But if we administer the life force abundantly present in flower essences to any living thing, watch the results.

Spirit-in-Nature Essences are based on the initial interpretations of the master teacher, Paramhansa Yogananda. Although to my knowledge Yogananda never made flower essences, he did list the psycho-emotional nutrients of the different fruits and vegetables from whose blossoms our essences are extracted, according to the methodology of Dr. Edward Bach. Commissioned by J. Donald Walters—a disciple of Yogananda for over 60 years and my friend and teacher—I developed these Spirit-in-Nature Essences in 1977, the oldest flower essence company outside the United Kingdom.

For nearly four decades, we have received testimonials and case histories, compiled through research and analysis, from people in the United States and overseas who have been significantly helped by Spirit-in-Nature Essences. Clearly, these infusions have the power to raise the quality of life for all living things—plants, animals, children of all ages, and we ourselves as living blossoms.

The *Essential Flower Essence Handbook* was first published in 1996. Since then, the acclaim for these essences continues to grow, along with a revised definition of the concepts I had developed up to that point—theme and plot applications and a few of the essences themselves. Also, the affirmations in this revised edition have been rewritten by J. Donald Walters, with my deep gratitude.

The concept of theme essences developed in Chapter Eight has also undergone some revisions, a theme essence being our predominant positive quality. Earlier editions of this book state that a theme remains constant throughout our lives. Now it's described as changeable, since we express different character strengths throughout our lives. This is a truer and more inspirational system to work with.

Lastly, Almond Essence, formerly for self-control and calmness, has the added dimension of *moral vigor*, for rebounding from setbacks in life. Apple Essence, described earlier for healthfulness, has been expanded to a new definition of *peaceful clarity*, a quality that supports health on all levels, especially in our attitudes. Also, Orange Essence, previously for joy, is now defined as *enthusiasm for life*. It's more accurate to say that joy can only come from within us.

Spirit-in-Nature Essences help us awaken to our highest potential. May this book assist you, and others through you, in attaining that goal.

The Essence of Life: Theme Song

Lila Devi

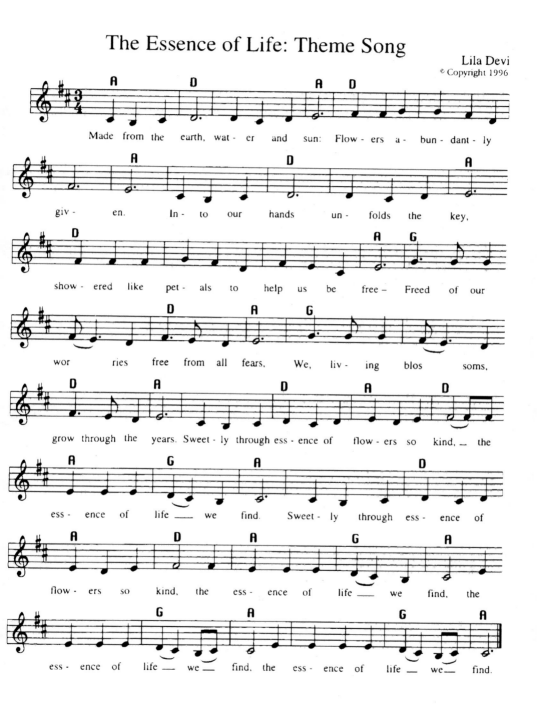

PART I

CHAPTER ONE

THE CONSCIOUSNESS
OF FLOWERS

"May you live all the days of your life." —Swift

"Life is pain, Your Highness," said the swordsman to the princess in a recent film, "and anyone who says otherwise is selling something." He was correct, in a sense, wasn't he? It's true that we live in seriously troubled times. If it isn't earthquakes, hurricanes, and other natural disasters, there are plenty of the man-made kind—rampant crime, drugs, and the pervasive decay of the family unit in the form of divorce, dysfunction, and abuse. To add to the list, we are now subjected to the madness of terrorists toying with highly sophisticated chemical weapons and the devastation of incurable viruses. Our present day culture is rent with chronic nervous tension, incessant instability, massive political unrest, and increasing violence. Adults and children alike—who among us is safe anymore?

There is hope, and that hope lies within us all—in our ability to change and to uplift ourselves. This, truly, is our task in life. And this is exactly what flower essences can help us to achieve. In the words of a modern-day saint: "Change no circumstance of my life; change me." Consider, too, this timeless message in the crypts of Westminster Abbey on an Anglican Bishop's tomb (1100 A.D.):

"When I was young and free and my imagination had no limits, I dreamed of changing the world. As I grew older and wiser, I discovered the world would not change, so I shortened my sights somewhat and decided to change only my country.

"But it, too, seemed immovable.

3

"As I grew into my twilight years, in one last desperate attempt, I settled for changing only my family, those closest to me, but alas, they would have none of it.

"And now as I lie on my deathbed, I suddenly realized: 'If I had only changed myself first, then by example I would have changed my family.'

"From their inspiration and encouragement, I would then have been able to better my country and, who knows, I may have even changed the world."

Our challenge being to change and uplift ourselves, where do we begin? What tools are at our disposal? As children, we go to the mother for comfort. As adults, we can still return to the bosom of the mother for nourishment and answers to our ills—our Mother Nature and the loving remedies that she proffers to us so abundantly through the plant kingdom.

Flowers are conscious, intelligent forces. They have been given to us for our happiness and our healing. This unique form of herbalism called flower essences is a concentrated encapsulation of pure life force, readily at our disposal. Herbalism has existed since the first human being prepared teas, tonics, and poultices—or even earlier, when the first wild animals instinctively grazed on plants designed to heal their wounds. In fact, even in this century, herbs are relied on as the basis of medicine. Today, twenty-five percent of all prescription drugs are derived from natural plant substances.

Flower essences, remedies, or drops as they are sometimes called, might also be considered "metaphysical herbs," because they work on a beyond-the-physical level of our being. Think for a moment about the power and beauty of flowers—their ability to cheer, to inspire, to comfort. Births, birthdays, illnesses, weddings, funerals—all are significant life experiences traditionally accompanied by bouquets of flowers. "Look at the flowers with critical insight," suggested Yogananda. "How could the flower evolve unless there were intelligence there?"

Likewise, we can hasten our own evolution through employing the tools offered to us by a conscious, caring Mother Nature—flowers and their essences. It has been humorously suggested that if everyone in the world gave one other person a back rub, all wars would cease. Translate this to everyone giving someone else a flower essence, and what do you think might happen? Let's find out, shall we?

CHAPTER TWO

THE EVOLUTION OF
FLOWER ESSENCES

"A human being is a part of the whole called by us the 'universe,' a part lim-ited in time and space. He experiences himself, his thoughts and feelings, as something separated from the rest, a kind of optical delusion of his conscious-ness. This delusion is a kind of prison for us, restricting us to our own personal desires and to affection for a few persons nearest to us. Our task must be to free ourselves from this prison by widening our circle of compassion to embrace all living creatures and the whole of nature in its beauty."

—Albert Einstein

VIBRATIONAL HEALING: A BRIEF HISTORY

The pharmacies and physicians of our age offer us a veritable buffet of healing modalities from which to choose when the need arises—or in preventive healing, *before* that need occurs. Depending on the nature of the illness and personal healing preferences, any modality from surgery to color therapy may appeal to us, from matter-oriented to energy-based treatment. Traditional allopathic medicine—an example of matter-oriented treatment—focuses on killing the specific disease, as in the use of antibiotics for infection or decongestants for the "com-mon" cold. Allopathy also treats specific organs once their function-ing is impaired, as in the many miraculous forms of heart surgery now routinely performed. What we call *vibrational therapy* deals with a strengthening of our entire psycho-physiological being by directly activating our life force. Thus are we granted a greater immunity to ill-ness and a higher quality of life. These two paths of healing need not conflict. Both have their place in the greater scheme of this universe, as described above by Dr. Albert Einstein.

Now let's trace the evolution of consciousness in the healing arts, woven thread-like throughout history, prefacing the appearance of flower essences. Hippocrates (c. 470-400 B.C.), considered the father of Western medicine, said, "Our natures are the physicians of diseases." This simple statement summarizes the philosophy of holistic medicine and provides the foundation for homeopathy, developed by Samuel Hahnemann (1755-1843). Homeopathy, meaning "like heals like," is based on the law of similars, much the same as today's vaccines. Hahnemann would give his patients a minute amount of a potentized herb or substance that, in healthy individuals, would cause the very disease that he was attempting to cure. Results were consistently positive. Evolved from this concept of using a small amount of poison to heal the poison within us, flower essences work with positives. Absorbing Nature's pure message through the essences can stimulate qualities that lie dormant within our own nature. In this non-invasive and painless manner, flower essences draw forth our own innately beautiful qualities.

Hahnemann also worked with the Doctrine of Signatures, an integral part of flower essence therapy as well—the concept that herbs are given to us through Nature's conscious design to heal the body parts that the herbs, in physical appearance, resemble. The plant's shape, color, scent, taste, and growth patterns all give clues to its healing use for our mental natures as well. But most important of Hahnemann's contributions was the principle of treating the patient and not the disease, according to Hippocrates' wisdom, to effect a true and lasting healing. This meant treating the "mentals," as they were then called, or personality characteristics, rather than the existing physical complaints—in other words, harmonizing the patient's psycho-emotional self so that his own conscious life force could act as the healer. ("Physician, heal thyself.") In a sense, this is the basis of flower essence philosophy.

Similar to homeopathy, flower essences do not directly treat the physical body or its symptoms. From a spiritual level, they address mental and emotional imbalances that, if left unresolved, eventually settle in the soil of the physical body, sprouting as physical symptoms.

As conscious beings who are aware of these subtle truths, we become the navigators of our own healing. Basically, flower essences are a response to the call of an ever-awakening humanity to minister to its spiritual needs.

A SECRET PHARMACY

When we trace back through the history of healing, we see two trends emerging: (1) a gradual shift of focus from matter to energy—in other words, from physical medicine to vibrational healing; and (2) the understanding that we can heal ourselves. Flower essences incorporate both directions of thought. They work by *bringing us into a state of harmony and resonance with our true essence—our internal perfect, or higher, Self.*

Mother Nature's pharmacy has long been accessible to those who have pried open her botanical medicine chest. And to those who wish to learn her language—the language of flowers—she bestows her most wonderful secrets of perfect well-being.

CHAPTER THREE

SEERS, SAGES AND HERBALISTS

"And now, here is my secret, a very simple secret: It is only with the heart that one can see rightly; what is essential is invisible to the eye."
— Antoine de St. Exupery, *The Little Prince*

The inspiring lives of herbalists Bose, Burbank, and Carver are testimonials that plants have conscious intelligence, feelings, and an ability to appreciate and respond to their environment. Dr. Carver called the plant kingdom an invisible world, one whose language everyone can learn—"if only they believe it." We too, believing, can fathom the plant kingdom's secrets of wholeness.

A BENGALI SCIENTIST

At the turn of the last century, Jagadis Chandra Bose made discoveries about the plant kingdom that were clearly ahead of their time. Perhaps it's for this very reason that his greatness went virtually unrecognized. Through construction of the crescograph—a sensitive instrument that microscopically measured the growth of living things—he confirmed that plants have a nervous system. He also found that they express a wide range of emotions, including love, hate, excitability, shock, fear, pain, and pleasure. With ultra-sensitive instruments, he was able to detect that insectivorous plants possess digestive organs similar to those of animals and that leaves respond to light, much like the functioning of the retinas of animals. Furthermore, he was able to measure in plants that had frozen to death a shuddering response similar to a death spasm experienced by animals.

It was Dr. Bose who first measured the phenomena that we call "metal fatigue," proving that metals, as well as plants and animals, are prone to exhaustion, overstimulation, and depression. In other words, *they too are conscious life forms.* An article in a British publication documenting his discoveries includes an experiment on vegetables, in which he concludes:

"Thus can science reveal the feelings of even so stolid a vegetable as the carrot."[1]

In his own words, Bose asks:

"Is there any possible relation between our own life and that of the plant world? The question is not one of speculation but of actual demonstration by some method that is unimpeachable. . . . The final appeal must be made to the plant itself and no evidence should be accepted unless it bears the plant's own signature."[2]

A California Botanist

"The secret of improved plant breeding, apart from scientific knowledge," said Luther Burbank, "is love." Nicknamed "the wizard of horticulture," Mr. Burbank reveals in this statement the simplicity and humility with which he made the most astounding discoveries. An American plant breeder born in 1849, Mr. Burbank explained that he would simply talk to the plants and create for them a safe, loving space. Through this unorthodox method, he was able to "encourage" a desert cactus to drop its thorns. "You have nothing to fear," he comforted the plant. "You don't need your defensive thorns. I will protect you."

By developing a deep communion with the plant kingdom, Mr. Burbank entered into their world to improve upon common flowers, fruits, and vegetables and thus eliminate their undesirable characteristics. With ease, he created new varieties of plums, berries, lilies, roses, apples, peaches, quinces, nectarines, potatoes, tomatoes, corn, asparagus, and numerous other plants. His name itself, Burbank, has become a verb listed in the dictionary that connotes improvement through selective breeding, as in the crossing or grafting of plants. The Burbank Gardens are preserved to this day in Santa Rosa, California.

AN ALABAMA AGRICULTURIST

The American herbalist, George Washington Carver, was born in 1864 of a slave mother. Through his utter simplicity and devout love of nature, he turned the tides of farming. He too had a nickname—"Black Leonardo." Dr. Carver discovered three hundred new uses for the peanut—previously considered useful only as hog food—and one hundred and fifty uses for the sweet potato, including coffee, axle grease, printer's ink, and cosmetics. Once asked how he uncovered the immense possibilities of these two common foods, he replied, "You have to love it (them) enough. Anything will give up its secrets if you love it enough. Not only have I found that when I talk to the little flower or to the little peanut they will give up their secrets, but I have found that when I silently commune with people they give up their secrets also—if you love them enough." [3]

In this description of a walk taken with Dr. Carver, one of his friends—who had intended to cover several miles in a few hours—wrote that they "did not get much farther than a hundred yards. At every little flower he met he had to kneel down. He examined it, caressed it, studied it, talked with it. This love of flowers of Dr. Carver has a lilt about it and a creative, living quality that comes only when love opens up to joy. People who love something to the point where love breaks forth in little fountains of ecstasy, are the ones who possess the secret of *par excellence*. And that is the degree with which Dr. Carver loves. . .with a love compounded of joy." [4]

THE PLANTS SPEAK FOR THEMSELVES

An extraordinary book, *The Secret Life of Plants* by Peter Tompkins and Christopher Bird, was published in the early 1970s. Were this text not backed by numerous documented experiments, it would read more like a fanciful fairy tale. One such story chronicles a cactus plant subject. Recorded through equipment much like what the Japanese police use for lie detection tests, the cactus produced song-like sounds with varied rhythms and tones. The sounds, amplified by electronic equipment, were reported at times as "even warm and almost jolly." This same cactus was also taught to count to twenty and perform simple addition, also registered by its sounds.

Not only do plants sing, but they are fully capable of musical appreciation as well. Sound waves, it seems, produce a beneficial effect upon plant cells, favorably influencing their metabolic processes. One of the more fascinating experiments reported in *The Secret Life* tested the effects of both classical and rock music on summer squash. The "subjects" were placed in structures much like glass aquariums. Light, temperature, humidity, soil, and water were all precisely controlled. One group of squash was exposed to Beethoven, Brahms, and other classical masters. These squash not only grew toward the source of the music, but one even entwined itself around the radio! The squash exposed to heavily accented rock music, on the other hand, grew in the opposite direction of the music. They even climbed the glass walls in what looked like attempted escape! This group—all with improperly developed leaves—either remained stunted in its growth or grew abnormally tall.

As an aside, I can't help being reminded of a testimonial from a woman in Dallas about her plants' response to an early recording of my songs about the flower essences. The songs blended vocals, instrumentation, and nature sounds that were apparently very pleasing to her potted friends. "My plants started blooming when I began playing the music. My African violet hadn't bloomed since I got it a year and a half ago. It sprouted baby buds—the rose geranium too." Who knows—perhaps the plants blossomed in celebration of their kingdom being musically honored! The point here is that all living things respond to being acknowledged, respected, and treated with kindness.

THE LANGUAGE OF FLOWER ESSENCES

Throughout recorded history, plants have set the stage for the drama of life. The legendary Sioux Indian medicine man, Black Elk, declared:

"For the Great Spirit is everywhere: He hears whatever is in our minds and hearts, and it is not necessary to speak to him in a loud voice." Likewise, Ayurveda, a six-thousand-year-old East Indian healing tradition, tells us that:

"The seers, through the yoga (union) of perception, let plants speak to them. And the plants disclosed their secrets—many of which are far more subtle than a chemical analysis could uncover. To become a true herbalist, therefore, means to become a seer. This means to be sensitive to the being of the herbs, to commune in receptive awareness with the plant-light of the universe. It is to learn to listen when the plant speaks, to speak to the plant as to another human being, and to look upon it as one's teacher." [5]

In keeping with herbalism's ancient traditions of communing with the plant kingdom, flower essences have evolved as a natural expression of healing—in the simplest ways, through the simplest means. "There are certain things," said Dr. Carver, "often very little things, like the little peanut, the little piece of clay, the little flower that cause you to look within, and then it is that you see into the soul of things." [6] Flower essences allow us to see into the soul of things—into ourselves, our world, and all living beings.

In the next chapter, we will take a glimpse into the lives of two remarkable men whose ideas cross-pollinated to breed a variation on a theme. Their transcription of Mother Nature's flowery song became Spirit-in-Nature Essences.

CHAPTER FOUR

THE ORIGIN OF SPIRIT-IN-NATURE ESSENCES

"Flower in the crannied wall,
I pluck you out of the crannies,
I hold you here, root and all, in my hand,
Little flower—but if I could understand
What you are, root and all, and all in all,
I should know what God and man is."
—Alfred Lord Tennyson

A physician and a metaphysician, living at the same time on opposite sides of the world and probably unbeknownst to each other, inspired the living roots of Spirit-in-Nature Essences.

THE MEDICAL MAGICIAN

The life of Dr. Edward Bach, founder of the Bach Flower Remedies, spans a mere fifty years—1886 to 1936. Considered a genius by his colleagues, Bach was a medical doctor, a homeopath, and a keen observer of human nature. Although he is generally credited with being the first to discover flower essences, it was the Swiss sixteenth century physician and alchemist, Paracelsus (see Blackberry Chapter Twenty-five under *Famous Theme Personalities*), who presaged Bach. Paracelsus recorded collecting dew from blossoms—the method from which flower essence preparation evolved—and administered it to his ailing patients.

Bach's was a sensitive spirit, attentive to the suffering of humanity and the bountiful healing blossoms of nature. Possessed of an abhorrence of the hypodermic needle, he sought a different means to relieve

the suffering of his patients. Dr. Bach eventually left his highly successful London practice to develop flower essences, leaving for us this
legacy—a healing art that was painless, inexpensive, and available to
anyone in need.

THE MAGNETIC METAPHYSICIAN

In 1893, seven years after Bach's birth, Paramhansa Yogananda
was born in Gorakhpur in northeastern India. A teacher and yogi,
poet and scientist, mystic and inventor, he arrived in Boston in 1920.
The youthful Yogananda was the first Indian yogi to spend his lifetime in America, lecturing in the States until his passing in 1952. His
spiritual classic, *Autobiography of a Yogi*, is published in over two
dozen languages. Inspiring small crowds to audiences of thousands,
Yogananda taught everything from meditation techniques (food for
the soul), to proper diet (food for the body). He found a keen hunger
in the American spirit for scientifically-proven techniques for self-
improvement.

Shortly after his arrival in America, Yogananda befriended Luther
Burbank—to whom he devoted a full chapter and the dedication
page of his autobiography. The two companions shared an ability to
perceive the divinity in nature, wearing their wisdom like comfortable
robes. Speaking of his gentle friend, Yogananda wrote:

"Behold a man in whom there is no guile! His heart was fathom-
lessly deep, long acquainted with humility, patience, sacrifice. His little
home amidst the roses was austerely simple; he knew the worthless-
ness of luxury, the joy of few possessions. The modesty with which he
wore his scientific fame repeatedly reminded me of the trees that bend
low with the burden of ripening fruits." [7]

In addition to his love of nature and beautiful settings, Yogananda
spoke in depth about many subjects relevant to health and healing,
including the principle of magnetism. We may understand that magnetism in the human body works very much on the same principles
as in physics. Consider a steel bar magnet in which all the molecules

are turned in the same direction, their north-south polarity aligned. Accordingly, *we* become more magnetic when our energy is aligned and without conflict. This principle of magnetism is strongly operative in flower essences that vibrationally align us with the positive qualities we seek to uncover within ourselves.

EVOLUTION OF SPIRIT-IN-NATURE ESSENCES

In a similar vein to the findings of Dr. Bose, Yogananda explained that food has consciousness. The fresher its quality, the stronger its *prana* (a Sanskrit word for life force). Thus the food we eat plays a part in shaping our mentality. Yogananda listed the psychological and spiritual qualities of different foods. Eat these foods and you ingest their "vibrational vitamins" as well—the peacefulness in pears, the enthusiasm in oranges, and the quiet dignity of strawberries.

If the cherry fruit contains a vibration of cheerfulness, think how much more concentrated is that quality in the cherry blossoms themselves! Botanists concur that flowers, being the reproductive system of the plant, contain ninety percent of its life force. Instead of utilizing the bark, roots, stems, and leaves as in traditional herbalism, Spirit-in-Nature Essences are prepared from the *blossoms* of the plant. Organic fruit orchards and vegetable gardens indigenous to the Sierra Nevada Foothills provide the blossoms for our essences, with the exception of Coconut, Avocado, Banana, Date, and Pineapple Essences that are made on the lush Hawaiian islands. The essences are prepared in such a gentle way, so respectful of the living plant that their life force is captured in the process. Flowers are plucked at their peak of ripeness; the plant itself is left intact.

In our culture, we speak so often about human potential. Bookstores abound with self-help books and life-enhancing workshops have become quite popular these days. Yogananda praised Americans for this very spirit of enthusiastic willingness. "Eventually, eventually," he said, capturing this spiritual essence, "why not now?" This is also the message of Spirit-in-Nature Essences. Why not live in our fullest potential *now?*

QUALITIES OF SPIRIT-IN-NATURE ESSENCES

Almond: Self-control, Moral Vigor

Apple: Peaceful Clarity

Avocado: Good Memory

Banana: Humility Rooted in Calmness

Blackberry: Purity of Thought

Cherry: Cheerfulness

Coconut: Uplifted Spiritual Awareness

Corn: Mental Vitality

Date: Tender Sweetness

Fig: Flexibility, Self-acceptance

Grape: Love, Devotion

Lettuce: Calmness

Orange: Enthusiasm, Hope

Peach: Unselfishness

Pear: Peacefulness

Pineapple: Self-assurance

Raspberry: Kindness, Compassion

Spinach: Simplicity, Guilelessness

Strawberry: Dignity

Tomato: Strength, Endurance

CHAPTER FIVE

THE ESSENCE EXPERIMENT:
A BIOFEEDBACK BRAINSTORM

"The greatest discovery of any generation is that human beings can alter their lives by altering their attitudes of mind." —Albert Schweitzer

MONITORING OUR "FLOWER FRIENDS"

In May 1996, Dr. Jeffrey R. Cram (now deceased), a clinical psychologist and nationally acclaimed biofeedback pioneer, conducted studies on Spirit-in-Nature Essences—the forerunner of many subsequent trials. The nature of the experiment: to see if individuals given their correct essences would demonstrate a scientifically measurable response to them. A single-subject design comprised this pilot study. This type of study means, simply, that individuals were compared with themselves and not with other groups of people. Thus, an experiment of this type is accurate even with fewer case studies.

Seven individuals were monitored. We used an A/B design on five of the subjects, which meant observing any changes in moving from point A to point B, with an intervention between the two points—in this case, administering an essence. This design measured a seven-minute baseline, or resting, stage; administration of a flower essence, determined through kinesiology just prior to the experiment; and observation of five minutes of response time. With two of our subjects, we added a third variable, creating an A/B/C design—a baseline, administering a brandy placebo, recording the response and then giving the actual essence followed by monitoring the essence response. (Please see the diagrams at the end of this chapter that profile both an A/B and an A/B/C design.) During all stages of the experiment, the subjects were instructed to remain silent and relaxed.

CHARTING THE PSYCHOPHYSIOLOGICAL

Our subjects' responses to the experiment were monitored by using transductors, or electrodes, placed directly on the skin at designated sites, using biofeedback equipment, also called "psychophysiology monitoring apparatus." These electrodes measured six signals, or response indicators, from the physical and metaphysical bodies. Two of these signals registered reactions in the physical body—hand temperature (blood flow measurement), and the EDA (electro-dermal response, or "skin talk," indicated by increased sweat gland activity). Monitoring the hand temperature traced the peripheral blood flow in the body. To explain, we are "internally wired" in such a way that if, for example, a saber-toothed tiger were to come charging toward us, the blood in our skin would be shunted away from the skin and into the muscles to make us stronger. If we tore our skin while fighting the tiger, we wouldn't bleed as much due to this protective, or survival, response. Hence, a cooling response in hand temperature in our experiment would suggest that the sympathetic nervous system is receiving more stimulation.

Sweat gland activity is a complicated signal, indicating an orienting response. We increase our EDA when we encounter something novel or that possesses a high signal value, such as hearing our name being called out. In other words, it helps us orient ourselves to the world. In terms of our tiger metaphor, an EDA response favorably adds more moisture to our skin, making it slippery and thus reducing the probability of tearing. Skin sensitivity is also increased, an aid in any fight-or-flight condition. In other words, if you were wired up to a biofeedback monitor and given an essence, and then registered an increased EDA response, we would say that the essence caught your attention, somewhat like a "wake-up call." Physiologically, you are responding to, and resonating with, the flower essence. For all seven subjects in our study, the EDA was the most sensitively responsive system in the physical body.

MAPPING THE METAPHYSICAL

The remaining response indicators, or EMG activity (electromyography), are derived from four of the *chakras* (a Sanskrit word meaning, literally, *wheels*, or centers of energy radiating from the astral spine): the third eye, or point between the eyebrows; the throat chakra; the heart chakra (not the physical organ); and the lumbar chakra, opposite the navel. Chakras, or energy centers, are those sites in our non-biological self from which health or disease radiate out into our bodies. Each center is associated with specific organs, located near the areas of the body where they reside. Particular qualities and emotions also correlate: the third eye, to joy and will power; the throat, to calmness and expansion; the heart, to love and intuition; and the lumbar, or solar plexus, to the seat of fiery self-control.

How is it possible, you might ask, to measure the metaphysical, or etheric, body scientifically? We might consider our experiment in terms of a study of new physics—no one has ever actually seen a quark or an atomic particle. Experiments on atoms are conducted in smoke, or cloud, chambers. Since researchers never see the particle, they look for the *trail* that the particle leaves in its wake. Similarly, our study monitored the trail, or measurement, of the change in metaphysical energy of our subjects. We do not literally "see" metaphysical energy, except through Kirlian photography that illuminates the aura, or magnetic field around the body. Rather, we see its footprints.

UNCOVERING THE ANCIENT SITES

In all of our subjects, we observed substantial changes during the first three minutes after administering the essence. On the following pages, you will see complete sets of six graphs for two of our subjects. Each vertical bar represents one minute. This simplifies in visual terms for the layperson how the physical and metaphysical bodies respond to the essences minutes after they are given, also strongly indicating that benefits are immediate.

Dr. Cram concluded: "The evidence from this pilot study clearly supports that flower essences do have an effect on the physical functioning of the body, the largest effect being measured in how we orient ourselves to the world through the EDA. In addition, this strong EDA skin response—an excellent measurement of the autonomic nervous system— reflects the interface between the physical and non-physical, or etheric, bodies. Flower essences also affect what I call the 'ancient sites' of the chakras, most notably the third eye. The lumbar center, for most of our subjects, was a strong responder as well. This part of the etheric body is also the origin point of *chi*, the term for life force in Oriental medicine."

Our two placebo subjects experienced no EDA response to the brandy placebo, but showed an enormous sweat gland response once the essences were administered. (They did register a strong response to the brandy placebo at the throat chakra, possibly from the warmth as it trickled through the physical throat—which is why we have eliminated the throat chakra signal findings as a definitive indicator in our study.) We deduced from this variable and from definitive responses in the lumbar, or *chi*, center, that flower essences do indeed measurably activate the life force, creating a resonance with it. The strong EDA response suggests that this awakening of energy, or "inherent, internal force," as Luther Burbank describes it, actually filters down to the physical body, confirming a significant response to flower essences. And from the third eye response, we can infer that flower essences raise what we might call, rather unscientifically, our "joy level."

How, then, do flower essences work? Very well indeed.

SUBJECT BR: A/B DESIGN

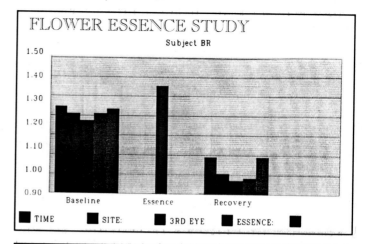

Third Eye: An enormous, striking response*

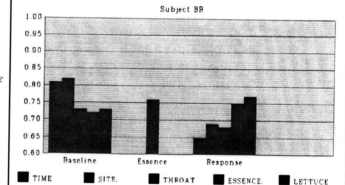

Throat: A small initial response of no significant duration

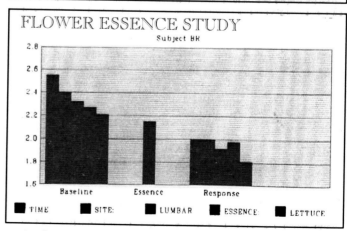

Lumbar: No significant effect here

* = Strong experimental effect

SUBJECT BR: A/B DESIGN cont.

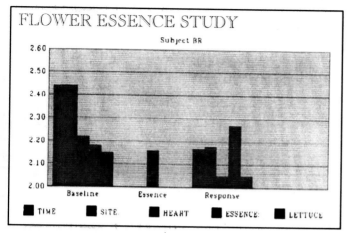

Heart: Only two points that are low, no consistent change

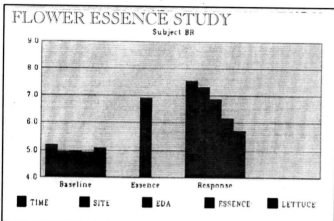

EDA: Flat, stable response, followed by an enormous jump in response to the essence*

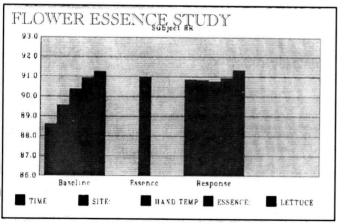

Hand Temp: Non-indicative response

* = Strong experimental effect

Third Eye: Diminishing response to placebo, marked response to essence *

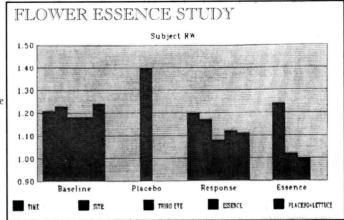

Throat: Both brandy placebo *and* the essence affect the throat *chakra*

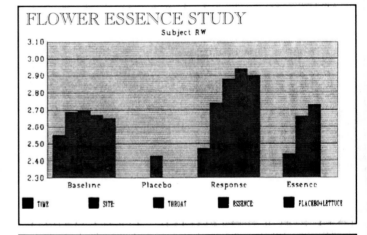

Lumbar: A flat reading on the placebo with the actual essence strongly activating this center *

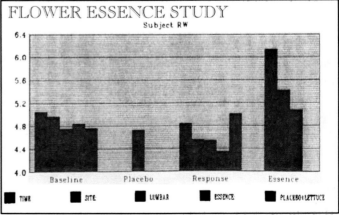

* = Strong experimental effect

SUBJECT BR: A/B/C DESIGN cont.

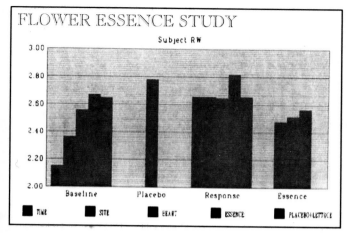

Heart: A stable response to the placebo; a nice quieting effect after the essence

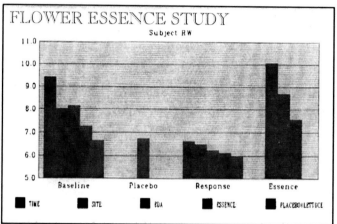

EDA: No response to placebo, yet a strong sweat gland activity in response to the essence*

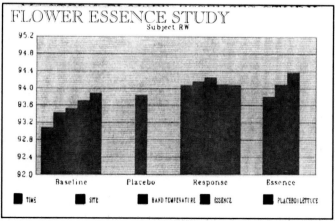

Hand Temp: Remains stable and thus non-indicative on both placebo and essence

* = Strong experimental effect

CHAPTER SIX

How Flower Essences Work

"Pray for a good harvest—but continue to hoe."
—Billboard at an Arkansas Baptist Church

The Active Ingredient

"I was playing out the same things over and over in my mind for months," recounted Stephen of a difficult breakup. "Now it's over and done with. The essences really allowed me to let go of what I was holding onto and release the pain." With the assistance of flower essences to vibrationally remind us of *who we already are,* we can break the false hypnotism of our human frailty.

Through the high vibratory rate of the blossoms from which they are prepared, flower essences interact with our *willingness* and *commitment* to change ourselves. Willingness and commitment equal *energy,* the active ingredient that we contribute to flower essence therapy. The essences activate our life force, the true source of healing. They work as catalysts, or pump-primers. For this reason, we may rightfully take credit for the changes that we co-create through taking the essences. A common response to them is, "Something's different, and I do feel better!" Or, "I really feel like myself again." Since happiness is our natural state, our desire to return to it, likewise, is only natural.

Energy generates magnetism, a subject that I mentioned in Chapter Four. A stronger magnetism vibrationally influences a weaker one. Consider this example: Handshaking is a way of transmitting magnetism, since our hands are actual magnets of energy. If a strongly negative person shakes hands with a weaker positive person, the weaker person will be negatively influenced.

Flower essences work in a similar fashion—*the essences, as living vibrations, both possess and project magnetism.* Their magnetism, being stronger and more positive than ours when we are out of balance, elevates us to their level when we "shake hands" with them. The essences work much like being in the presence of someone who inspires and uplifts us. In taking the essences, we place ourselves in their "presence."

In the journey we undertake with flower essences, we are lifted up to their higher rate of vibration. A musical metaphor can also illustrate this point. A flower remedy may be likened to a tuning fork. By attuning ourselves to it, we become in tune with the song of our unique perfection. With the essences, we look to balance and thus strengthen our life force. And since each individual is different, there is no pat formula or set order of essences. Each essence program is as unique as the person following it.

Will the changes initiated by the essences last? People often ask this question. In most cases, the answer is yes—although none of us are immune to backsliding! As a rule, it's also true that we heal in stages, attaining deeper levels of clarity over time rather than categorically clearing lifelong issues instantaneously. If you take Raspberry for forgiveness and expansiveness of the heart, you may experience a response similar to Stephen's, mentioned earlier. The change will most likely be permanent, *provided that your thoughts and actions continue to support it.* If, for example, you take Tomato Essence to gather the strength and will power to disentangle yourself from a contractive relationship, it will not be in your best interest to return to that unhealthy situation. Environment, it has been said, is stronger than will power.

An Essence for Everyone?

Are there remedies for everyone? Yes! For anyone—including plants, animals, and children. Basically, the remedies can help *anyone* or *anything* with life force. This sounds a little too good to be true, doesn't it? You might ask, what about the mother-in-law on heavy antidepressants or the intimidating stray tomcat who seem completely disinterested in self-improvement? Well, personally, I would rather err on the side of giving *everyone* the benefit of the doubt. Since flower essences, at worst, would only be ineffectual, why not let the in-law and the old tomcat at least try to better themselves? If they *still* refuse to "get their act together" on essence therapy—well, at least the effort was made. (As a reminder, flower essences do not replace proper medical attention, nor are they recommended as such.)

Why should we give everyone the benefit of the doubt? Because we needn't even be aware of our desire to change in order for the essences to help us. That very energy is what activates the essences to work for us. This is why skeptics make excellent flower essence clients—at least they are putting out the energy to question what flower essences are all about! Let's assume that no one, animals and plants included, wants to be miserable. When we are not expressing the truth of our higher self, we are not happy. Darkness and darkening qualities must, by their very nature, someday fall away from us. *They are not us.* We are not the negative habit patterns that we sometimes express. These patterns, like surface dust on a fine sculpture, have no real existence of their own beyond the recognition we give to them. Our conscious desire to grow in positive directions, supplemented with flower essences, can virtually annihilate them. It is to our credit—and our healing—to remain non-identified with our flaws and to view them dispassionately.

WELL, THEN: AN ESSENCE FOR EVERYTHING?

In a delightful scene from the stage play "Fiddler On The Roof," the townspeople ask the village rabbi if there is a prayer for everything. In response to his answer in the affirmative, they plead, "Rabbi, is there even a prayer for the Czar?" Momentarily meditative, he responds in full cantor's voice, "May God bless and keep the Czar. . .far away from us!" Wild applause erupts.

Often clients ask, "Is there an essence for everything?" "Do you have an essence for my husband's procrastination?" "My sister-in-law is so overbearing—what do you have to make her change?" "Which essence works for insomnia?" "My son is teething—is there an essence for his discomfort?" A generic answer is, yes, there is an essence for everything. Implicit in our desire to be restored to wholeness is the remedy itself. True seeking leads to sought-after answers.

Enter Flower Essences

Now, back to the above questions. Although Corn addresses procrastination and Grape is wonderful for bossiness, the real issue at hand may not be other people, but *us*. (To clarify: throughout this book, the capitalized plant or food name refers to the actual flower essence.) Our strength lies in our ability to work on *our* issues and confront our own tailor-made tests. In truth, we are powerless over others except to the extent that we project a positive magnetism, inspiring them by our example. And what victory when the shortcomings of others no longer negatively affect us! Considerable self-honesty is necessary in order to realize that the flaws we see in others may be exactly the ones that we ourselves possess. If we find bossiness in someone else, it would be worthwhile to introspect on whether we, too, harbor that tendency.

As for the second set of questions above—yes, Lettuce can help with *the emotional states* causing the insomnia, and Orange is helpful for teething pain in the same way. Flower essences work with the energy that triggers these physical issues, not directly on the actual physiological states. When peace of mind is restored, any latent seeds of illness may remain unnourished and thus unable to sprout. Sometimes, however, illness is necessary for our spiritual growth, offering us needed lessons. In these instances, we needn't look at illness or even death as failure. *Flower essences do not remove our tests; they help to clarify them.*

To simplify, all flower essences do the same thing, for every living thing—*they restore us to a state of balance in which our internal, intelligent life force is activated.* Life force is the real healer; the energy of the flower essences merely primes it. The uplifting qualities embodied in flower essences are our truest nature; our task is to access those qualities.

WHAT FLOWER ESSENCES DON'T DO

Essences do not affect us biochemically, as does traditional allopathic medicine. Sedatives, for example, can knock you out for the night. This is not the case with flower essences. In other words, they *allow* us to change; they do not *make* us change.

Here's an important point: *flower essences will not change us into anything but our true selves.* Thus we never need worry about misusing them to manipulate our own or other's behavior. It's simply not possible. There's a joke about a man who, upon having his arm set in a cast, asked the doctor if he would be able to play the piano when it healed. "Of course," replied the doctor. "Good!" said the man, "I couldn't before." This is not the case with flower essences. Without altering our essential nature, they allow us to refine who we already are.

CAUSE FOR CRISIS—OR CELEBRATION

Let's talk now about the phenomenon known as the "healing crisis." Often, people believe that, in order to heal, toxins need to be flushed out of their systems, either physically or emotionally. Granted, when strong emotions or repressed abuse issues are finally allowed to surface, they may pour forth like a veritable tidal wave. Here, the practitioner's sensitivity is called into play to support the client's healing process, without either stifling or magnifying it by interpreting it as a crisis. A good practitioner can help the client understand that he is not being given more than he can handle, with the knowledge that issues surface only when we are ready to deal with them. Yes, we may be stretched beyond what we *thought* we could endure. But is that not how we grow? (As an aside, you'll see the masculine singular used in this book, i.e., "someone/he," as traditionally written, rather than the grammatically incorrect and genderless "someone/they," that is off-putting to the English major in me. I ask your tolerance—there is no chauvinism intended.)

I propose replacing the term "healing crisis" with "awareness celebration." The release of the most painfully buried memories can be accompanied by an even deeper joy. This is the joy of freedom: liberation from stored pain and growth from acknowledging that the truth of who we are is, and always has been, untouched by that pain. Flower essences in and of themselves do not draw out emotional toxins—*they merely make us more aware.* In nearly 40 years as a flower essence practitioner, I have seen only a handful of people experience a true "healing crisis." In each case, the individual was energetically ready for a breakthrough at that point in time and could just as easily have undergone a catharsis from chewing bubble gum!

Paradoxically, there are practitioners who report that most of their clientele experience the classic "healing crisis." Is this attributable to the essence line, the practitioner, or the client's identification with a crisis rather than a celebration? Indeed, individuals often report energetic breakthroughs on their essence programs in the form of insights, clarity, fresh realizations, and the breaking of old patterns that no longer serve them. Shall we label this process a crisis, or celebrate it as our release from mental and emotional blockages? One practitioner explains, "My experience is that Spirit-in-Nature Essences do not pull you through all your emotions. You don't go through the drama—the issues just fall away."

IN ESSENCE

There are two basic schools of thought in the field of healing: one, that it requires as long to cure an illness as it took to acquire it; the other, that of flower essences—that we can change in an instant, much like turning on a light in a darkened room. Physical and mental imbalances, according to Yogananda, spring from one, and only one, illness—ignorance of our true nature that is perfection. "The reason people's lives are so dull and uninteresting," he explains, "is that they depend on shallow channels for their happiness, instead of going to the limitless source of all joy within themselves."

Many people, by choice, live on the periphery of their consciousness, only skimming the surface of true joy. Just the other day, the trainer who checked my membership card at the health club asked, "How ya doin'?" "Oh, fine," I replied, "and yourself?" "Just great. It's Friday and I'm really going to party tonight," he continued, with a significant commitment of energy behind his words. Parties end; true happiness born of the commitment to simply *be* happy does not. Flower essences help us awaken to that limitless source of inner joy. And how do we reach that state? Through healthy, balanced living and the gentle assistance of these essences that *vibrationally remind us of our own perfection*. It is by realizing our inner perfection, in this moment, that we tap into that joy.

SPIRIT-IN-NATURE ESSENCES SPECTRUM

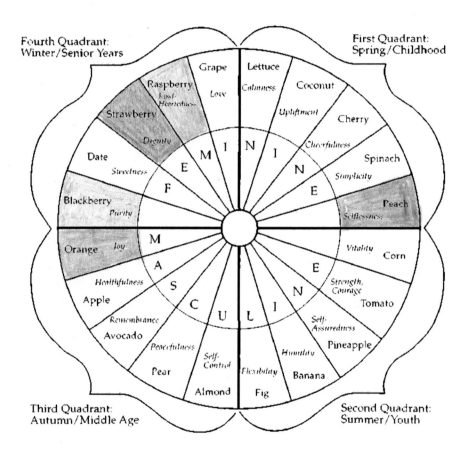

CHAPTER SEVEN

To Everything
There Is a Season:
The Spectrum

"When I walk with you I feel as if I had a flower in my buttonhole."
—William Makepeace Thackeray

The rational part of the human mind loves charts, diagrams, and systems of classification. They can give us clarity, context, and a sense of order.

We have the sun/moon/ascendant in Western astrology; vata/pitta/kapha in Ayurvedic treatment; and rabbit/monkey/snake in Chinese astrology, as but a few of the systems we use to try to understand ourselves! For this reason, I hope you will enjoy these next two chapters (and Chapter Thirty-one), whether you are an essence novice or a well-versed practitioner. They are intended to explain Spirit-in-Nature Essences in a workable system, though are in no way meant to limit the whole of humanity with finite definitions.

THE ESSENCE SPECTRUM CHART

A spectrum is, literally, "a series of colored bands diffracted and arranged in order of their respective wave lengths, by the passage of white light through a prism." The word, *prism*, stems from the Greek, "to saw," and refers to "a solid figure whose ends are equal and parallel polygons and whose faces are parallelograms." I have chosen this name for our chart because a spectrum describes a series of colored bands, more commonly called a rainbow, which is a symbol of hope.

And hope is the underlying message of every flower that ever graced the earth. Also, color is vibrational, as are the essences. In a sense we too might be considered prisms, as beings of light that diffract qualities, somewhat like colors, into the different facets of our personalities.

This Essence Spectrum Chart, then, provides a thematic overlay of Spirit-in-Nature Essences. It is neither necessary nor recommended to take them in this particular order. Nor is it true that only women can take the ten feminine essences or that only children can use the remedies in Quadrant I—although taking the former can help us to develop our feminine nature and the latter, our childlike side. The Spectrum maps a directional flow of energy, explaining how the essences can lead us on a journey of self-discovery.

We could say that this journey, one essence-step at a time, represents the maturing process of the personality. Opening like blossoms, we learn our life's lessons. Just as no two flowers are exactly alike, so also are no two human beings identical. Our journey, then, is a progression—not in terms of specific years, but of a flow of consciousness. In this chapter, we will examine the ways that each essence thematically evolves out of the one before it and into that which follows. Accordingly, each essence symbolizes a gathering of wisdom, happiness, and inner freedom on our path toward realizing our highest potential as human beings.

The essences may be likened to pieces of a stained glass mosaic, each with a different shade and texture—opaque to clear, smooth to beveled—which comprise the totality of our unique personalities. Your expression of Strawberry's dignity, for example, will differ from anyone else's. Your closest friend will express the kindness of Raspberry in ways very different from your own.

The Essence Spectrum Chart is divided into halves according to predominantly masculine and feminine essences and into Quadrants representing life stages and seasons of the year. This chart, then, illustrates the flow of nature's cycles with stages of life. It proclaims, as do all ancient healing arts, that we are a part of a greater universe, consciously created.

Two Halves

Quadrants I and IV comprise the feminine half of the Spectrum. The ten essences grouped here possess qualities that are more feminine in nature—yielding, inward, inspirational, receiving, nurturing, and basically feeling-oriented. Quadrants II and III constitute the masculine half. These ten remedies contain qualities that are more masculine—outwardly expressive, driving, building, creating, achieving, and reason-oriented. Flower essences as living energies possess both male and female attributes, much as we do. In ways similar to us, they are predominantly either masculine or feminine. For example, Pineapple contains the feminine qualities of inwardly knowing oneself, and inspiring others through that knowledge. It also outwardly expresses the more masculine qualities of confidence and competence. The latter qualities—necessary tools for success, especially in the business world—being dominant, Pineapple is located in the masculine half of the Spectrum.

Four Quadrants

The Spectrum is also divided into four Quadrants of five essences each, representing the seasons of the year—spring, summer, autumn, and winter. It also symbolizes the four basic stages of life—childhood, youth, middle age, and senior years. Each Quadrant also depicts a complete cycle within itself. If we decide to strengthen the youthful side of our personality, we would look to the Quadrant I essences in the Spectrum; for more ripened, mature, and inward qualities, we would study the fourth Quadrant.

The First Quadrant

In Quadrant I, we find essences that capture the qualities of springtime and childhood—Lettuce, Coconut, Cherry, Spinach, and Peach. Spring heralds the completion of winter when living things begin to grow again. Having hibernated under the snow, plants and animals now bask in the sun's warming, life-affirming rays. Shadows, along with daylight hours, lengthen in a symphony of awakening greenery and the newborn of many species take their first breath.

The first Quadrant also symbolizes that period of life that includes birth, infancy, and childhood. As new arrivals on this earth, we make acquaintance with our parents and siblings. We grapple with attempted mastery of our bodies—walking, talking, eating, tying shoes, and eventually taking the training wheels off our bicycle. Exploration, excitement, and wonder abound in the Quadrant I essences. These five essences also reside in the feminine half of the Spectrum. Not yet weaned from the mother figure, they exemplify the qualities of adaptability, softness, gentleness, and receptivity.

Lettuce, the first essence in this Quadrant, represents the personality at birth as a clean slate, or a calm mind. From this vantage point, we are now ready to be filled with direction, creative endeavors, and the making of choices. Coconut is the white chalk with which to write on this slate. The hallmark of Coconut is expansiveness; it conveys the ability to see the whole picture and live more in a superconscious, solution-oriented state of mind.

Through this uplifted state, we find ourselves in tune with a positive energy flow—the cheerfulness epitomized by Cherry. Cherry is the child skipping, hopscotching, and seeing the bright side of every circumstance. Cherry's good cheer evolves into Spinach. Playful, full of wonder, undaunted, and trusting, Spinach represents the fully nurtured little one. The functional Spinach child then matures into Peach, the caregiver. Peach, Quadrant I's final essence, is also the transitional remedy into the next Quadrant. Peach represents an embracing of others and a concern for their needs, signaling a shift of focus from the self to others in preparation for moving into Quadrant II.

THE SECOND QUADRANT

The second Quadrant contains essences that express the fire of summertime and youth. The summer season recalls images of a more intense sun, greens parched to paler shades, longer days, and clear night skies. To the young, this means a time to party; to stay out late, test their strength, and rebel with a newly formed will power, growing into a sense of "I-ness." "Gather ye rosebuds while ye may," lyricized romantic poet, Robert Herrick, "old time is still a flyin'. For this same flower that smiles today, tomorrow will be dyin'." If, in truth, youth is wasted on the young, it's a fact to which they remain blissfully oblivious!

Comprising this Quadrant are Corn, Tomato, Pineapple, Banana, and Fig. In the masculine half of the Spectrum, these essences all express a predominantly male energy—moving forward in life, owning one's power, and energizing the ability to accomplish tasks.

Corn, the rambunctious offspring of Peach, sends energy moving with a wave of raw vitality. "I can!" it affirms, "I can do anything, when so I think!" What better way to charge through life than bursting through our fears with untimorous Tomato. Also called "the warrior essence," Tomato's strength leads us to the self-assurance of Pineapple. Fearless and invigorated, we develop self-knowledge and trust of that inner wisdom.

Lest it become self-inflated and proud, Pineapple is now tempered by Banana's humility, with its ensuing calmness reaped through non-involvement and detachment from life's countless ups and downs. Balancing Banana's attitude of non-attachment, we move on to Fig, for flexibility and self-acceptance. Fig addresses rigidity of the body and mind. It ensures that our ideas about ourselves and the world around us do not limit, calcify, or constrict us.

The Third Quadrant

Flexible, malleable, and strengthened by the lessons of Quadrant II, we now pass into the third cluster of essences for autumn and middle age, completing the masculine half of the Spectrum. Here, we reap the wisdom thus far acquired on our journey. Perhaps we find ourselves in midlife crisis, questioning the choices we have made. Maybe our career has reached its peak of fulfillment. Maybe our work in the outer world is nearing completion, and we find it's time to redirect our energy toward more interiorized pursuits. The children, if we had them, have now grown and gone, giving us the space for a more contemplative life.

In autumn, we harvest our garden of character strengths so carefully planted a short while ago. The earth's life force, chased by the dropping centigrade, withdraws into its core. Leaves, now paper-like and multicolored, waft to the ground, escorted by colder breezes. Tree limbs wax brittle. Animals in the wild prepare for the coming winter, just as we prepare for this ripened stage of life.

Quadrant III includes Almond, Pear, Avocado, Apple, and Orange, consecutively. Opened through Fig, we are now ready to be tempered by self-control, moral vigor, and the moderate use of our senses dictated by wisdom rather than whim—Almond. A harmonizing calmness ensues through Almond's message of living the courage of our inner convictions.

Emerging from the negative state of that calmness—unruffled, unmoving—is the messenger of the perfect peace of Pear. Peace of mind, that most valuable commodity, is the stepping stone to remembering our purpose in life—Avocado, for good memory. "Ah, now I remember!" says Avocado.

In recalling that *raison d'être*, we may realize that we have always been well and whole. Peaceful clarity is our birthright, and the missive of Apple essence. Apple's expression of healthy attitudes manifests as the enthusiasm of Orange. No matter how deeply rooted our sorrows may seem, Orange washes them away, leaving us with the sweetly pungent taste of inner bliss.

THE FOURTH QUADRANT

We now embark on the fourth and final Quadrant of winter and senior years. This Quadrant echoes sweetness, resolution, and completion. The muted, dried browns of a withdrawn autumn are now blanketed in the feather comforter of winter white. Snow and ice, like advancing years, slow us down, entreating us to bundle up and tread carefully over a snoring earth. Rhythms slacken while the days, like half-burnt candles, wane. And we, again like children in this season of maturing years, become more dependent on others. Thus, we return to the feminine half of the Spectrum with a well-ripened maturity and a storehouse of inner riches.

Quadrant IV contains Blackberry, Date, Strawberry, Raspberry, and Grape. From a spirit made radiant through Orange, we turn to Blackberry. Like a cleansing snowfall, Blackberry's message purifies us with clean thoughts, honesty, and honest self-assessment. Blackberry allows us to see the goodness in ourselves and in those around us. These qualities make us sweet and without judgment—the lesson of Date. Harboring this tender sweetness, we draw the same to ourselves, magnetizing the company of family and friends to our side, thus enriching the winter of our lives.

All too often, winter is likened to decline or decay when it is merely the cycle preceding spring. In Strawberry lies the first hint of approaching rebirth through the ennobling quality of dignity. Mature, refined, and stately with the accumulated wisdom of the years, it bespeaks a certain softness, much like a perfectly ripened strawberry.

Only when we value ourselves can we truly value others. Here the seeds of Raspberry for kindness sprout into wondrous heart qualities of empathy, sympathy, and true sensitivity to others. In forgiving those who have deeply hurt us, we reap great benefits, including the ability to forgive ourselves. Healed of our own emotional wounds, we are then able to help others do likewise.

The Spectrum, like the astrological Aquarian, pours its life-giving waters into the final essence—Grape—for unconditional love. Grape's is the love that liberates instead of binds; the love that seeks to give rather than to receive; the love that is its own fulfillment. Selfless love wells up not from any outer source, but from the center of our being that longs to love. Love is the truest healer. Love is the comforter. Love is the essence of life.

GOOD HEAVENS

To everything there is a season, we are lovingly told, and a time for every purpose under heaven. The Essence Spectrum Chart provides a time and place, philosophically speaking, in which to develop our inner strength and beauty.

CHAPTER EIGHT

THEME AND PLOT ESSENCES

"Be thou thine own home, and in thy self dwell." —John Donne

METAPHORS AND MEANINGS

This chapter serves to explain a new terminology for the world of flower essences—theme and plot applications, when to use them, and how they are determined. Basically, flower essences fall into two categories, of theme and plot essences. This means that we each have one theme essence, with occasional exceptions, and nineteen plot essences within the context of the 20 Spirit-in-Nature Essences, all coming into play at different times in our lives.

To simplify, we could say that we face our life challenges in one of two ways: (1) we remedy a negative quality by replacing it with its positive opposite; or (2) we build on existing strengths. The first approach summarizes the work of plot essences; the latter of theme essences. For example, Joseph, as we'll call him, had a stressful day at work, and so he returned home and took Spinach as his plot essence, to help him simplify his life. Margaret also had a difficult day, but decided to take her Peach theme essence because it reinforced her compassionate nature. This essence allowed her to be impervious to the day's difficulties. Both individuals selected essences that helped them return to their own core of inner strength, and to deal more effectively with life's infinite daily challenges.

THEME ESSENCE

It has been said that the entirety of a person's life could be encapsulated into a movie of a couple hours' length. Imagine yourself as a feature film at the local cinema. In what category of the movie reviews would you be listed—comedy, drama, musical, action/adventure, or family entertainment?

Isn't this a playful thought? On a deeper level, though, you may find clues to your theme essence. In literary terms, we have the word, *theme*. A theme is defined as the thread of conflict through which we struggle to discover ourselves—our strengths, our shortcomings, and just-who-are-we-anyway. This conflict may take any of these forms: man-versus-man, man-versus-nature, or the more philosophical man-versus-himself. It is through these frictions in our lives that we sculpt the masterpiece of our spiritual growth.

A theme essence refers to a dominant positive quality in our personality. It is that quality in which we are particularly strong; the one we resonate with; the one we closely resemble. In classic homeopathy, a theme essence would be called a constitutional; in flower essence therapy, a *type* or *personality remedy*. It is interesting to note that in traditional flower essence therapy, a type remedy is determined according to one's overriding negative or unperfected characteristics—which is our definition of a pivotal plot essence, explained later in this chapter. A Grape theme, by *type remedy* definition, would be someone who is typically domineering and ruthless. However, according to *theme essence* constructs, a Grape theme is someone who is predominantly loving and devoted.

Hence, our theme essence is the one that addresses a major recurring theme or quality in our lives. We have, to a great extent, already mastered this quality but are always applying the finishing touches. Our theme essence issue is one that we return to again and again, working on deeper and more refined levels over time. This means that we draw to ourselves the very tests we need to resolve corresponding issues in order to attain perfection of that quality—or at least to aspire in that direction!

Let's look at our Grape theme again. He may draw to himself the loss of parents or dear friends early in life. "What does this mean?" he is forced to question. Later on, perhaps divorce triggers this need to understand love on deeper levels. Or loneliness may recur. "What is this human suffering trying to teach me?" he asks again. Until he can answer these questions, he will continue to attract custom-designed outer circumstances that will afford repeated opportunities for understanding. Thus he will magnetically draw certain tests through his need to experience love's true nature, which is the lesson of Grape.

The degree to which we express the perfected nature of our theme essence is reflective of our personal evolution. For example, the more we exhibit Almond's self-control, the more we will express its perfect state of balance. Also, the more refined our consciousness, the more difficult it becomes to pinpoint a theme essence. We may express the unconditionally loving Grape and also emanate Pear's perfect peace of mind. At this point, all the essences blend together. In this way, we grow through the vibrational support of flower essences.

One further note: since the theme essence is intrinsically linked to the personality, it can often be masked by personality-altering states such as mental retardation, diseases such as Alzheimer's, and psychotropic drugs, both prescription and recreational.

EXAMPLE OF A THEME ESSENCE

Let's examine the life of Helen Keller and her corresponding theme essence. Born in 1880, Ms. Keller lost the senses of sight and hearing at the age of nineteen months. Through the efforts of her loving teacher, Anne Sullivan Macy, she learned to comprehend the connection between words and objects and, at ten years of age, achieved a major victory—speech. In her twenty-fourth year, she graduated *cum laude* from Radcliffe College. Ms. Keller authored six books, and became the subject of several films, including the adapted Broadway play in 1959 entitled *The Miracle Worker*. She is also noted for her valuable contributions to the American Foundation of the Blind as counselor on international relations.

Even without experience in intuiting theme essences, we can see that Ms. Keller's was a life of unmitigated courage, strength, and the overcoming of obstacles. These are the hallmarks of a Tomato theme.

Faced with extraordinary barriers to the natural abilities of the senses that most of us take for granted as commonplace, she fought time and again to master the simple art of the spoken and written word. Even the titles of her books suggest the courage and will power of her undaunted spirit: *Optimism* (1903), *Out of the Dark* (1913), and *The Open Door* (1957). "Life," she professed, "is either a daring adventure—or nothing." Ms. Keller's life, indeed, exemplifies that of a warrior. The message of Tomato permeates her heroic courage in the face of immense obstacles.

THE FLOWER/FOOD CONNECTION: THEME ESSENCE

"I *love* 'real' cherries, though not in cough syrup or pies," confesses a Cherry theme. "I adore almonds—I eat them every morning for breakfast without fail," admits an Almond theme. "When I do eat pineapple, I really enjoy it, especially in jello salad—but doesn't everyone?" asks a Pineapple theme.

You get the picture. We have a special relationship with the food that corresponds to our theme essence. In nearly four decades of consultations, I have grown accustomed to asking clients how they react to their theme essence food. Gradually, a pattern has revealed itself. Ninety-five percent of the time, people express a particularity, and a peculiarity, toward the food that corresponds to their theme essence. Here is a sampling of theme essence food stories:

"Oh, tomatoes—love them, especially the cold Beefsteak variety. I love to wear that color—the richest, ripest, most sun-drenched shade."

"I like coconuts, though I don't eat them a lot. But I love coconut milk, especially on oatmeal. I love it *fresh*. I like it, I like it!"

"I love fig preserves—though fresh figs are decadent! Fig seems like a fruit for a king."

"I even wear strawberry perfume and use strawberry shampoo!"

"Raspberries are my favorite food group. I could live on them! We've got some great ones growing here. I buy six flats and freeze them so I don't run out during the off season."

"I live on asparagus," someone volunteered at one of my classes.

"Does this make me an Asparagus theme?" Well, obviously our system includes only the twenty Spirit-in-Nature Essences, and the whole of humanity most certainly won't fit into this finite system! For now, however, it's the one we have to work with. Also, we need to substantiate a theme essence with more than food cravings. They are, unquestionably, important clues—though like a good Sherlock Holmes, be sure to collect more evidence!

How to Determine Your Theme Essence

Sometimes others can see our theme essence more clearly than we ourselves do. Why? Because we are too close to ourselves. Distance, perspective, and self-honesty are necessary in order to decipher our own theme. A friend of mine who is an excellent Spirit-in-Nature practitioner, thought that she was a Blackberry theme. She values her ability to analyze and introspect as paramount. A runner, yoga teacher, and massage therapist, she often expresses a clarity of purpose. This individual whom we would playfully call a "health nut" had Apple practically shouting to be acknowledged as her theme essence!

To determine your own theme essence, you might ask yourself, "Am I really *that* peaceful, or *that* clear-thinking?" You might also spend time with true themes of the type you suspect yourself to be and see whether your energy matches theirs.

Above all, trust yourself. You will spot a Pineapple from a Pear theme a mile away—though distinguishing Pineapple from Corn may take some work. Watch for the feelings people evoke in you to determine their themes—it's a simple issue of magnetism. A Pear theme will draw forth your own inner peace; a Pineapple will renew your innate self-confidence. And remember that the voice and eyes give us excellent theme essence clues, since they both reveal and project magnetism.

Try the following exercise to decipher your theme essence. With pen and paper, take some time to answer the following questions. Be thoughtful but also spontaneous in your answers. Your first thoughts will most likely be the most revealing. This exercise may be used for

family, friends, and clients in order to determine their theme essences
as well.

1. The qualities I most admire in others are. . . *friendliness / kindness / presence*
2. The outstanding idiosyncrasies of my personality are that I . . .
3. The main qualities I am trying to perfect in myself are . . . *humility*
4. It really bothers me when other people . . .
5. The three adjectives I would use to describe my energy are. . . *high / positive / chaotic*
6. If my life could be ideal, what I would change is. . .
7. Am I calm? Kind-hearted? Cheerful? (pick the quality of a theme essence you suspect.)
8. Do I like and sometimes crave spinach? Grapes? (or whatever food corresponds to the theme essence in question.) *banana*

Are you still caught in the "doubting Thomas syndrome?" Here's a little game I like to play to sharpen my theme-detective skills. While waiting in line at the checkout counter, the airport, the DMV, take a moment to observe people. Study them, breathe them, intuit them. Spinach themes are very straightforward in nature. Pineapples will draw your attention—to themselves or their actions. It's easy. Before long, you'll be an expert!

"I don't want to be a Corn theme, I want to be a Peach!" shouted a client at the end of our consultation in a very loud, Corn-theme voice. "I'm really not a Raspberry theme," one woman announced, "I'd much rather be a Strawberry." What to do? Well, first it's helpful, and honest, to admit that no one is infallible, including the practitioner. Do bear in mind, though, that discerning your own theme is not as easy as deciphering other people's themes. Secondly, there is absolutely nothing wrong with being a Corn theme. Each essence has its own innate strength and beauty. And as we aspire toward our state of perfection, the distinctions of the essence definitions fade. Lastly, if you'd rather be a Peach then a Corn theme—be one! Theme essences are not set in stone—we can aspire toward whatever qualities we wish to develop within ourselves.

On a grander scale, countries have personalities and thus themes as well. To some extent, we are tempered by the temperament of our homeland. Fun-loving, childlike America is a true Spinach theme. A scene from a recent movie comes to mind of a man touring his friend through a prestigious part of Los Angeles. "Some of these homes," he proclaims, "are over twenty years old." Impressive! Then there's the will-oriented Tomato-theme Germany; the carefree and somewhat careless Cherry-theme Mexico; the devotionally loving and passionate Italy, our hallowed Grape. This can be food for thought when planning your next vacation. (As to a country's inevitable plot essences, well . . how about Pear, "the peace-bearer," for times of warfare and natural disaster; Orange for *economic* depression, followed by Pineapple to internally empower the country and restore its consciousness of abundance; and Tomato for the courage required to simply read the newspaper headlines!)

In addition to a theme essence, some individuals have a sub-theme essence. This is similar to having a major and a minor in college—both are predominant areas of study with one having a greater focus of energy. Examples follow in some of the essence chapters under *Famous Theme Personalities*. To summarize, a sub-theme is a lesser though still significant theme.

Lastly, it's okay to guess wrong. It is better to try and fail than fail to try!

PLOT ESSENCES

Now on to plot essences and back to our literary metaphor. Plot refers to the path followed throughout a story. The plot may take many turns. Since the plot implies action, movement, and thus energy, we would employ plot essences where different issues, problems, or tests arise that require our attention. Here, unlike the theme essence, we see the negative indications of an essence surfacing—nervousness requiring Pear, immoderation wanting Almond, rigidity leaning toward Fig. The term "negative" does not imply dark, bad, or wrong. It merely suggests a lack, or absence, of the positive quality, as in photographic negatives where the light and shade of a subject are reversed.

Plot essences are straightforward. Are you studying for an exam? Avocado. Are you working too late and too often? Almond. If you find yourself feeling out-of-sorts, select the essence that can help you to return to your natural state of balance.

Plot essences are divided into two categories—*pivotal* and *peripheral*. A pivotal plot essence is a strongly needed, recurring plot essence. Our pivotal plot essence may masquerade as our theme due to its predominance and our repeated need for it in our lives. The difference between the two is that the pivotal plot essence is indicated by a *lack* of expression of the desired quality, while the theme essence *strengthens an existing positive quality*. Both are indicated on a frequently recurring basis.

Consider, purely on a level of magnetism, the saying that opposites attract. Applying our new terminology, this means that we are drawn to friendships, and especially love relationships, with those whose theme essence matches our pivotal plot essence. Sara, for example, is a loving Grape theme. Also a mother of three and involved in numerous volunteer jobs, her pivotal plot essence is the energetic Corn which is her husband's theme essence. Sara finds herself drawn to other Corn themes for friends, since their Corn energy supplies her with "missing vibrational vitamins."

Here's another intriguing concept: theme/theme connections, or the "birds of a feather" syndrome. We are also drawn to people of our same theme essence, who are familiar and thereby comforting to us. Thus, connecting with others of our own theme is fortifying and reinforcing. To explore the match of a theme essence with a pivotal plot essence can be dynamically charged.

Now, on to peripheral plot essences. These include the remaining essences that surface as needed from time to time. "Gosh, I'm fuzzy today, I need Apple." Or, "I'm too caught up in this argument—where's my Banana?" Peripheral plot essences generally do not manifest with quite the same urgency or depth of need as pivotal plot essences. They are more surface-layered, or peripheral, to our nature. The difference between pivotal and peripheral essences is easily deciphered by both frequency and intensity. Because flower essences delight in breaking rules, there are always exceptions. Pear may be urgently indicated for accidents, for instance, or Lettuce for extreme emotional agitation.

EXAMPLE OF A PLOT ESSENCE

Madeleine worked in a gift shop in a small West Coast tourist town. She often found herself judgmental and impatient with customers and co-workers. After a week on Date, her pivotal plot essence indicated by a curt nature, she reported feeling more irritated than ever. Madeleine experienced a seeming setback, as if the essence had "backfired." We discussed this turn of events and decided that the problem had actually not worsened; her *awareness* of it had grown, a common reaction to flower essences. Two days later, Madeleine called with this news—her judgmental, easily irritated pattern of reacting to customers had dissolved and she felt more at peace with herself than ever.

FLOWER/FOOD CONNECTION: PLOT ESSENCES

We find the flower/food connection operative with both theme and plot essences, the difference being that plot essence foods surface less often than theme foods and tend to relate more to specific events.

"The week my divorce proceedings began, I ate nothing but oranges and bananas."

"I started craving tomatoes when I moved to the city."

"Every time I have a rough day at work, a fresh spinach salad really does the trick."

"I ran out of bromelain that I was taking for athletic overuse of the muscles and resultant inflammation. So I ate pineapple instead—one a day. I started feeling like a really bumptious, cocky, swaggering sort of person!"

"I have never liked peaches, but I started eating them during the breakup of my marriage. I had started thinking too much of 'me.' I ate lots and lots of peaches, and found myself getting really interested in other people and listening to them."

HOW TO DETERMINE PLOT ESSENCES

It's both simple and easy. The prerequisites are being in touch with your feelings and honestly assessing your needs. Above all, please remember that we want to identify negative traits, not identify *with* them. How can we determine our plot essences? By observing the discrepancy between how we are thinking and acting and how we want to be. By accessing the positive Coconut qualities within our nature, we can then assess the qualities we need to draw upon from within the storehouse of all our existing fine qualities.

THE ULTIMATE PARADOX

Assuming you've got the basic concepts down, try to grasp this concept—the rare person with the same theme and pivotal plot essence! Here we see an individual expressing both the strengths and weaknesses associated with a given essence in equal intensity. Gemma, for example, is an Apple theme/pivotal plot. She teaches hatha yoga, boasts of an impeccably clean diet, and actively inspires others to be more mindful of their own psycho-physical conditions. This same woman is herself always questioning herself, afraid of reliving the illnesses of her genetic family and filled with doubt about which therapies to explore for her own healing. Then there's Jake, an obvious Fig theme/ pivotal plot. Good nature and good humor are his positive Fig theme characteristics. Extreme fanaticism and rigidity around health issues are the negative. The magnetism he projects to others is indeed a mixed bag—inspirational with his noteworthy disciplines and repellent by an inferred sense of their own imperfections. So if you're sitting on the fence, metaphorically speaking, about a client's theme or pivotal plot essence, they could be one and the same.

"DOING" VERSUS "BEING"

To summarize, plot essences are symbolized by *doing;* theme essences, by simply *being.* Our theme essence is the framework on which plot essences are stacked. The theme essence signifies being at home; plot essences are the path we take to get there.

Consider Madeleine, described earlier, a Coconut theme (this was determined in the course of a consultation). We noted that her life revealed the repeated theme of tests that required great amounts of sustained, persevering energy and thus much inner growth as a result of finding superconscious solutions. Her Coconut "stick-to-it-iveness," in fact, helped her to remain on Date as a pivotal plot essence.

How do we know which essence to take at a particular time—plot or theme? As a general rule, plot essences work with negative states; theme essences, when things are going well but not quite well enough—or when theme issues arise. Taking our theme essence provides a special sense of comfort and familiarity, a sort of at-homeness. We might even say—when in doubt, try your theme essence. Our theme essence can, and does, change as different character strengths emerge, rather than remaining stationary throughout our lifetime.

To put it differently, our theme essence is the individuated way we express our divinity. And it is through this expression that we return to that divinity. We could also say that the flower essence is the vibrational quality, the theme essence is our expression of that quality, and the plot essence represents our need to express that particular quality.

Above all, remember there is no need to worry about your essence choices. Trial and error are our best friends. Fortunately, essence selection is not as serious as choosing a life partner, a matter in which Socrates lightly encouraged us not to worry: "By all means marry; if you get a good wife you'll become happy; if you get a bad one, you'll become a philosopher."

Theme and Plot Essences Identified

Flower Essence	A positive vibrational quality
Theme Essence	Our positive, dominant expression of that quality
Sub-theme Essence	A secondary positive expression
Plot Essence	Our need to express that particular quality
Pivotal Plot Essence	A frequently recurring need to express that quality
Peripheral Plot	A need expressed occasionally in specific situations

our need to express that quality

← plot → doing → work w/ negative states

theme → being
↳ taking provides a sense of comfort + familiarity

CHAPTER NINE

THE DOOR AJAR:
HOW TO USE THE
ESSENCE CHAPTERS

"He who has imagination without learning has wings but no feet."
—Fortune cookie

METAPHORS AND MAGIC

A flower essence is like a multi-faceted gem, each surface representing different subtopics under a single theme. For instance, Strawberry's theme is dignity. Issues of self-worth, maturity, and poise are but a few of its facets. I have attempted to reveal the dimension, color, and life of each essence in the following chapters.

These essence chapters have been a great challenge for me and an even greater joy. In the process of writing them, I've learned more than could be told in words. I have sculpted the essences in literary clay, as it were, interpreting them at greater length for the first time. Also, I have attempted to give them both wings and feet, that they might alight on the flowering of your own understanding. Rather than presenting definitive, all-conclusive statements that would only confine the essences in tiny, finite boxes, I have offered at times metaphors, stories, and famous quotes, somewhat like the literature from the Orient, that leaves the door ajar to further understanding.

Chinese writing differs from that of the Occident. It harbors a deliberate ambiguity—one that, paradoxically, seeks to clarify rather than to confuse. Instead of literally translating an experience by mere definition, the Oriental description of a healing art offers a parallel. It paints a picture and relates a parable. Take, for example, the acupuncture point named after a particular rock. There is a kind of rock, affording shelter from the wind, that juts up from a river. This story-scene is a metaphor for a particular turning point in our lives; symbolic of a crossroads, it refers to a time when decisions are made.

The information you are about to read is gleaned from nearly four decades of collected research. I hope this book, like the rock in the river, will be a turning point for you and a new beginning of a continuous stream of expanding awareness.

ESSENCE CHAPTER FORMAT

FLOWER/FRUIT/FOLKLORE

Corresponding to the flower illustration and the Latin description of each essence plant with its English translation, here you will find facts about the tree or plant from which the fruit grows as well as the blossoms themselves, and historical information about the plant's origins. Flower and fruit folklore abound through the ages, passed down from generation to generation. Humanity's innate wisdom authors these not-so-mysterious myths, catching their thread of truth through the tree, plant, flower, and fruit. Here also, you will find nutritional information and health benefits of the food sources.

QUALITY/MESSAGE/PATTERN (QMP)

This section refers to the *Quality, Message of Self-mastery,* and *Pattern of Disharmony* provided for each essence, offering a helpful essence summary. Its purpose is to give a brief introduction to, and synopsis of, the essence.

Quality: The essential nature of each Spirit-in-Nature Essence, summarized in a word or two.

Message of Self-mastery: The beneficial effect of the essence, resonating with, and thereby awakening, that quality within us; the vibrational quality of the essence.

Pattern of Disharmony: Indicates the need for a particular essence; a negative habit, i.e., weakness or imbalance, strengthened through repetition.

To summarize: the *Message of Self-mastery* is the essence quality that connects us to our own source of perfect well-being, and the *Pattern of Disharmony* is the ingrained habit that separates us from our inner joy.

SPECTRUM PLACEMENT

This brief section reviews the essence's Spectrum position in relation to those that precede and follow. It explains both the essence's individuality and its connection to the larger picture in terms of the Spectrum's Quadrants and halves.

POSITIVE APPLICATIONS

A text version of the *Message of Self-mastery*, this section explains the positive essence state. I have added stories, quotes and occasional humorous anecdotes where helpful. The *Message of Self-mastery*, *Positive Applications* and *Positive Expressions* sections together offer a more complete view of this positive essence state.

NEGATIVE INDICATIONS

The word "indication" simply means "the need for." We may understand this part of the chapter as an expansion of the *Pattern of Disharmony* section with examples, quotes, and direct testimonials added when appropriate.

The *Pattern of Disharmony*, *Negative Indications*, and *Negative Conditions* sections are all designed to present a picture of the need for a given essence from different angles. If they seem a bit on the harsh side, remember that we are working with degrees. Date's negative judgmentalism, for example, may manifest as a deeply critical nature or just a passing unkind thought. Remember that we want to identify negative traits, not identify *with* them.

THEME ESSENCE CHARACTERISTICS

You may want to refer back to the "Theme and Plot Essences" chapter as you study the next three sections in each of the essence chapters. I have devoted several sections of each essence chapter to the subject of theme essences because: (1) the concept and terminology for a positive type remedy are new and are virtually unpioneered in the flower essence world; and (2) understanding these themes will be an important part of your flower essence work with yourself and others.

The physical and psycho-emotional traits of each theme, plus the magnetism they project to others, are covered under this subtopic. Although the positive theme characteristics are explained here, please remember that we can also exhibit our theme's negative side, i.e., pushiness for Grape or absent-mindedness for Avocado. This simply means that we have not yet perfected our theme essence quality. The negative theme essence characteristics are identical to the plot essence indications, i.e., *Pattern of Disharmony*, *Negative Indications*, and *Negative Conditions* sections. Also, remember that these theme characteristics are generalizations. Not everyone with bowed posture, for example, is a Banana theme.

FAMOUS THEME PERSONALITIES

Here, I have listed several famous personalities who richly exemplify the different themes, profiling the first in detail. Our subjects include historical personages, presidents, scientists, fictional characters, heroes, heroines, saints, sages, movie stars, rock stars, and sports stars. Although it was not possible to interview the people listed here—since they were either inaccessible or long gone—I have assessed their themes from reliable literature either by or about them, and sometimes both.

CONFESSIONS OF A THEME ESSENCE TYPE

Having heard from the famous, I then added this section as a more informal sharing. In other words, if an essence had a voice, what would it say? Here, you will read a direct first-person account from each theme type, in his own words. In addition to each person's unique brand of charm, these theme individuals articulate their own levels of clarity about themselves. Their testimonies reveal a focus on both the positive and negative aspects of their theme essences. The Pineapple theme, for instance, dialogues her sense of insecurity, although she more than hints at a strong sense of self-knowing. Through these peoples' own words, we are given a bird's eye view of their strengths, their fears, and their stories. The individuals interviewed were not told their theme essence until the end of the session. During the course of the interview, they were asked questions similar to those in the theme and plot chapter under "How to Determine Your Theme Essence."

WRAPPING IT UP

To complete the text section of each chapter, several paragraphs tie together the salient points previously explained. I have also used this section to take the liberty of relating interesting folk tales or some-times to illustrate the Doctrine of Signatures that, in Spirit-in-Nature Essences, applies to the fruit as well as the flower, plant and tree. This summary section conveys a vibrational portrait of the essence in its entirety. Having been dissected in a sense, here it is put back together.

CONTRAST/COMPANION CHART

When two people join together, a third entity—their relation-ship—is created. Such is also the case when two flower essences pair off, as explained in this section. The first, or *contrasted essences* column, distinguishes those essences that are similar, parallel, or even seem to duplicate one another. Subtle yet definite differences set them apart. Paradoxically, these same pairs also make excellent *companioned essenc-es*, as shown in the second column. Companion essences are those that bond especially well with each other. You might say they vibrationally walk arm-in-arm together and can be taken in close proximity time-wise, i.e., finishing one and immediately beginning the next. Consider, for example, Almond and Tomato. These two essences are contrasted: Almond addresses self-control in overcoming immoderate habits and behaviors, whereas Tomato helps to battle addictions and, over time, eliminate them. Almond offers a completely different approach than Tomato toward overcoming obstacles—Almond, energetically inward and upward; Tomato, a straight-on approach. The two also make excellent companion essences because they apply to similar issues. When used in close proximity in time, they aid in the development of psycho-emotional health.

POSITIVE EXPRESSIONS

Here we find the positive qualities of each essence that we exhibit when acting in harmony with it, and thus with our true nature. This section, as in *Negative Conditions* below, lists the essence qualities in adjective form.

You will notice some overlap here of the same quality for several essences. For example, both Corn and Pear share the positive quality of willingness, though with slightly different expressions. Corn captures the quality of free-flowing, accessible energy; Pear's counterpoint is the willingness born of resolved conflict and/or resistance.

NEGATIVE CONDITIONS

This section overlaps the *Patterns of Disharmony* at the beginning of the chapter. What the *Patterns of Disharmony* section describes in phrases, the *Negative Conditions* section lists mainly in single adjectives. The latter is intended as a reference guide, or a mini-index. (See the appendices for the complete index.)

Please note: you will find some duplication of terms with the *Quality/Message/Pattern* description in both this section and the next. Each, however, has a different intent. The QMPs provide an overview of the essence to introduce the chapter, whereas the *Negative Conditions* and *Positive Expressions* sections are intended to be used as a handy, at-a-glance reference. The Grape chapter, for example, catalogues thirty-two negative indications—not to be elucidated in a book of this size! Also, some essences have shorter lists than others. This is no indication of their importance; they simply require fewer words. And remember that the presence of even one *Pattern of Disharmony* is reason enough to administer that essence.

ESSENCE ENHANCERS

The purpose of this section is twofold: (1) to offer supportive measures to supplement the essences you are taking; and (2) to support *you* as holistically as possible. In other words, instead of only taking the essences four or more times a day, experiment with the Essence Enhancers. They can help you to be more mindful of the issues you are working on. Taking action imprints needed lessons into our conscious and subconscious minds. The more consciously you work with the essences— *instead of expecting them to work on you or in place of you*—the more quickly and dramatically you will see results.

Some people even like to wear the color of the essence they are taking as a further reminder. Try eating more of the corresponding food as another way of tuning in to the essence. You may want to sample some of the recipes in the appendices as well.

Consider spending some time with theme essence individuals who are strong in the essence in your program. These living embodiments of particular essences provide us with examples of that essence's message. In the presence of Corn themes, for instance, we absorb their raw energy and enthusiasm; in Date themes' company, their contagious sweetness and acceptance of others.

Also, let common sense be your guide. Some Essence Enhancers apply across the board—proper diet, rest, and exercise for the body; a positive environment, an anti-stress schedule, and other self-nurturing measures for the mind; and meditation for the spirit. These activities, as well as the individual visualizations and affirmations, may accompany all of the essences, and thus are not listed specifically unless they especially enhance particular essences. Finally, listen to and sing your essence songs (see Products and Programs, page 345). These "aural affirmations" are imbued with the vibrations of their corresponding essences. You will also want to read and review the chapters about the essences you are taking. The chapters themselves are written with the vibration of their corresponding essences. Reading about Cherry may actually cheer you, whereas the Avocado chapter is intended to act as a "mental pencil sharpener."

Also, feel free to create your own "designer Essence Enhancers." This is basically a "whatever works" section.

VISUALIZATION

Visualization employs our faculty of imagination that, in Italian, is called *la fantasia*. Some people are better at this than others, perhaps because they are more visually oriented. This section acts as a sort of visual affirmation by conjuring a mental image, described as vividly and storylike as possible. Basically, it serves to get us out of our minds and into a *feeling* of the essences.

AFFIRMATION

Each essence is interpreted as an affirmation. Trying saying it as you take your drops. (See pages 269-270 for an explanation of affirmations and also our Affirmation Deck in Products and Programs, with more information on our website.)

THE SECRET HEART

I have attempted to write the following twenty chapters from within the secret heart of each essence. Acting as their interpreter, I have translated their unique vibrational articulation into the medium of words. No doubt, you will see in them a little of yourself, family, friends, and clients. Above all, don't get discouraged by imperfection! We are all on a journey toward Self-realization. At various stages in our lives, different essences will come into play. In time, with effort and grace, we will find ourselves expressing their radiantly beautiful qualities and becoming our own living blossoms in the process.

PART II

CHAPTER TEN

LETTUCE:

"THE UNRUFFLER"

Lactuca compositae ("daisy-flowered, milky")

"Thank you so much for Lettuce. I was much calmer during the presentations I've made recently." —*JH, Ft. Collins, CO*

"I took Lettuce hourly the day of, and then just before, giving a lecture. I felt totally calm in front of an audience of forty people. I was surprised at how relaxed I was!" —*SW, North San Juan, CA*

"My daughter would scream at night from eczema. After one drop of Lettuce on two consecutive nights, she fell back to sleep immediately both times. Also, I took one drop of Lettuce before a harrowing visit to the periodontist. I was instantly calmed." —*MS, San Leandro, CA*

"I use Lettuce to relax into sleep, for after meditating at night I'm often too charged up to relax. I use Lettuce, too, if there are uncalming things going on with others in the environment." —*RB, Bend, OR*

"My son is still waking up a lot at night, but on Lettuce, I am handling it better. I'm not as wound up as before." —*RS, San Francisco, CA*

"I felt a definite sense of peace on Lettuce—closer to my center. When you get sick, your energy scatters. It brought my energy more toward that center, and made severe facial poison oak easier to cope with." —*CS, Colfax, CA*

"The tempest is o'er blown, the skies are clear,
And the sea charm'd into a calm so still
That not a wrinkle ruffles her smoothe face." —Dryden

FLOWER/FRUIT/FOLKLORE

Considered one of the oldest vegetables, lettuce dates back to antiquity and supposedly originated in the Near East, Siberia, or the Mediterranean. All cultivated varieties probably stem from the wild prickly lettuce, an Asiatic weed. Lettuce belongs to the daisy family *(Compositae)*. When bolting, it produces an aged, flowering stem and bears small, pale yellow flowers. Leaf lettuce is more nutritious than head lettuce because the sun is able to penetrate each leaf. Rich in vitamin A and low in calories with a ninety-five percent water content, lettuce is excellent for weight loss. Lettuce juice can be used to promote sleep.

Quality: Calmness

Message of Self-mastery: Inner quietude; inner strength in confrontation of difficulties; clear communication skills; unblocked creative expression; success in undertakings; decisiveness; ability to speak one's truth; concentration.

Pattern of Disharmony: Restlessness; too many thoughts at once; inability to concentrate; excitability; troubled emotions; agitation; propensity toward anger; nervousness; inability to make decisions; repression; emotional congestion; repeats self in conversation.

SPECTRUM PLACEMENT

Lettuce occupies Quadrant I's first house. It contains the qualities of springtime and childhood—youthful exuberance, and the crispness of winter melting into the season of planting and rebirth. It is a time to begin anew and start afresh. Introducing the feminine side of the chart, Lettuce carries within it a softness and delicacy, a lightness and quiet interiorization. You will find in all five of the Quadrant I essences a certain simplicity of expression—a what-you-see-is-what-you-get quality.

POSITIVE APPLICATIONS

The positive Lettuce state is a joy to behold. Here we see the sailboat personality forging "full speed ahead" into creative projects such as writing, painting, woodworking, or calligraphy. In the performing arts, one in the positive Lettuce state breezes across that fine transition line between the actual creative process and its presentation before an audience. Thus we see the annihilation of the performing artist's most painful dilemma—stage fright. "Will they like me? Will my work, representing the essence of my being, be accepted?"

In a state of inner certainty, Lettuce offers the antidote to an indecisive mind. Remove the anxiety, fear, and attachment to the outcome of a decision, and we see an individual with all the knowledge—or the ability to gather it—needed to resolve most any problem.

On a less grandiose scale, the highest octave of Lettuce manifests as a calm mind. A great saint of South India, Thayumanavar, put it rather succinctly:

> *You may control a mad elephant;*
> *You may shut the mouth of the bear and the tiger;*
> *Ride the lion and play with the cobra;*
> *By alchemy you may earn your livelihood;*
> *You may wander through the universe incognito*
> *Make vassals of the gods; be ever youthful;*
> *You may walk on water and live in fire:*
> *But control of the mind is better and more difficult.*[8]

In the positive Lettuce state, we are able to speak up for ourselves instead of "stuffing it" when we feel mistreated. All too often, repression creates resentment and anger that can later manifest as emotional outbursts. Repression is also the host for snide comments that often become increasingly more difficult to trace back to their source. It is better to be "up front" and nip problems in the bud in the positive Lettuce state through the simple act of clear, direct communication. For example: "You know, son, it's a good idea to ask before taking the car in case Mom or I need it." Or, "I was really hurt when you made that comment about my hair. Can you explain what you meant?"

NEGATIVE INDICATIONS

The negative Lettuce state manifests much like a stampede of wild-horses running amuck with thoughts shooting out in several directions at once—or with emotions that do us harm, anger in particular. Of all human emotions, anger is probably the most destructive. It is actually known to destroy brain cells, not to mention causing deep agitation in each and every bodily system. An angry person breathes spasmodi-cally, aborting every attempt to feed oxygen to the body. It's best not to eat when angry; food is literally poisoned with indigestion-producing chemicals.

"I am convinced that Lettuce saved my marriage," wrote Simon. "I was about to strike my wife, but took Lettuce instead and calmed down instantly."

Restless thoughts and emotions can be likened to sediment stirred in a pond. In such a mental state, decision-making is impos-sible. Although individuals in the negative Lettuce state may be well informed and highly intuitive, it is possible that they will be unable to reconcile even the simplest decisions—such as what to order from a dinner menu! For this reason, they seek advice from sources outside themselves, perhaps investing in costly therapies. Or they may stretch the patience of their friends by wavering back and forth on decisions, finally spinning themselves into the ground with energy spent and answers unresolved.

What can we do with a mind that is not within our control? In the negative Lettuce state marked by agitated thoughts or emotions, suc-cess is virtually impossible. Attainment of even minor goals remains an illusive dream without the necessary ingredient of concentration; and concentration is the fruit of calmness.

THEME CHARACTERISTICS

Lettuce themes emote a soft-spoken voice with an interiorized tone, much like hearing someone speak from a distance, almost as if with a slight echo. They are very inwardly centered and seemingly withdrawn. These people speak their truth, though without Blackberry's outspokenness.

Like a wind through a forest, Lettuce themes touch the lives of many people and are thus very influential, though in an understated way. They possess great strength of character. They stick to what they believe in, and they express themselves clearly. In their own quiet way, they put people at ease in their presence. Being in their magnetism leaves you feeling relaxed, calm, and energized.

FAMOUS THEME PERSONALITIES

Henry David Thoreau
Ben Kingsley
Denzel Washington
Madeleine L'Engle
Walt Whitman
Stephen Foster
Joan of Arc
Albert Schweitzer
Kabir
Lao-tsu

Henry David Thoreau (1817-1862), our Lettuce theme, was the son of a pencil-maker and the gardener of his influential friend, Ralph Waldo Emerson. Thoreau's famous treatise on civil disobedience exemplifies a Lettuce theme who spoke his truth. He brought calmness to an arena of great unrest in troubled times fraught with unjust laws that usurped individual rights, including slavery.

Most famous for his book, *Walden*, Thoreau writes of the divinity in nature and its ability to put the human spirit at peace. He spent two years at Walden Pond in Concord, Massachusetts, drinking nature's calming influences, as a man who chose to "live deep and suck out all the marrow of life." Thoreau wrote that "most men lead lives of quiet desperation." His life, to the contrary, bore testimony to the quiet fulfillment of the Lettuce theme. True to his own writings, he forged a life in communion with the harmonious universal laws of nature. His example and his works have inspired other reformers such as Gandhi, Tolstoy, and Martin Luther King, Jr.

CONFESSIONS OF A LETTUCE THEME: ROSALYN'S STORY

"My childhood was pretty traditional—standard, Midwestern, middle class, mom and dad, four kids. Our family took a vacation every year, but we weren't real close, you know. It was average, I'd say. I was basically happy. When I look back, we just sort of went through life with nothing outstanding. It was a meat-and-potatoes family.

"I am manager of a small rural health clinic. I like the work because I'm a pretty mental person with lots of mental energy—always thinking, working on quieting my mind. Emotionally, well—I'm not real emotional. I'm basically pretty steady. I can get emotional but I tend to hold it in. If I do get emotional, I get mad inside, and don't express it. Am I calm? Generally, yes.

"I do like lettuce. I especially like to pile it on sandwiches, the crunchy kind—that taste! I can't have a sandwich without lettuce, and I really like salads. Any kind of lettuce will do, as long as it's crunchy."

WRAPPING IT UP

Lettuce, then, offers us the experience of strength, wholeness, and balance through the simple quality of calmness. When the subject of Lettuce's calmness arose in one of my classes, an older gentleman piped up, "Excuse me, I don't get it. How can you be calm and have energy at the same time?" Make no mistake—calmness is not synonymous with laziness! Laziness indicates a *lack* of energy whereas true calmness reflects an abundance of it. Pure energy, when focused, *is* calm.

With calmness of mind and thus of body, we can meet our challenges, both great and small; use our inner strength to deal with life's ongoing tests; and realize our creative potential in whatever unique ways we choose to express ourselves.

LETTUCE	Contrasted With:	Companioned With:
Almond	for calmness gained through control of the senses	being centered in oneself and respectful of what is needed to stay in balance
Banana	for calmness from stepping back from one's problems	to be an observer of one's own life and not get caught up in disturbing emotions
Blackberry	for negative or judgmental thoughts	for the pure discrimination of a calm mind
Pear	for a more general sense of well-being	to enhance the quality of calmness on deeper levels
Tomato	for fears of known and unknown origin (with the exception of stage fright)	for "calmness in the midst of battle"

POSITIVE EXPRESSIONS

Clear
Creative
Certain
Clear in communication skills
Quiet
Withdrawn in nature
Successful
Decisive
Able to speak one's truth

Concentrated
Patient in parenting
Healthy in interpersonal relationships
Trusting of inner guidance
Emotionally steady
Patient
Tolerant

NEGATIVE CONDITIONS

Restless	Unable to concentrate
Repetitive	Repeating failures
Emotionally congested	Excitable
Advice-seeking	Troubling, disturbed emotions
Thinking too many thoughts	Agitated
at once	Angry
Lacking in focus	Nervous
Scattered	Stagefright-prone
Vacillating	Repressed
Indecisive	Confused

ESSENCE ENHANCERS

Do the following breathing exercise: inhale, hold the breath, and exhale, each to a count of ten. Gradually increase to twenty-five counts.

Meditate.

Spend time alone.

Create a peaceful and inviting environment at bedtime with soft music, candles, an inspiring book of quotes or seed thoughts (I highly recommend the line of *Secrets* books by J. Donald Walters).

Take time to cultivate a postponed creative pursuit.

VISUALIZATION

Imagine yourself in a setting of pure tranquility. It is a calm, sunny spring morning and you are seated on the bank of a still pond. The water, a reflection of complete quiescence, is neither cloudy nor clear. What first strikes you is the absence of any breeze, the still life quality of nearby wildflowers, and the crispness of the artfully paletted hillside. Color is everywhere, bursting into myriad greens beneath your bare feet.

Now, see yourself merging with the scene before you, your very body dissolving and expanding into its environs. By an act of creative will, bring movement into this pastel still life—much as a composer would add different movements to a symphony—all the while maintaining a sense of complete calm. A bird glides overhead, the subtle song of its wings grazing the sky. A small fish peeks out of the glass-like layer of water that now splinters into a medley of ripples.

Motion without movement is a song without a single superfluous note. This is your self-portrait, painted with brush strokes of calmness.

AFFIRMATION:

I am calm. I am free. In undisturbed stillness, I find my true home.

CHAPTER ELEVEN

COCONUT:
"THE UPLIFTER

Cocos nucifera
("nut-bearing monkey")

"I woke up today saying, 'This is it—no more stress. Don't go to work.' I called in sick. Then I took Coconut and felt my spirits lift. I previously felt that the job—and the world—were on top of me. Coconut brought my energy from despair due to overwork to a sense of utter serenity, and that I would be taken care of."   —KA, Palo Alto, CA

"I took one drop of Coconut at the kitchen table. By the time I had walked over to the refrigerator, I actually felt taller. Hard to imagine since I am 6'4"! I felt euphoric for the next three weeks."

—CH, Los Altos, CA

"On Coconut, obstacles in my life became games that I felt I could easily win."   —SN, Charlotte, NC

"Taking the Coconut was truly amazing. If a remedy's going to do something, I'll feel it right away. My spine straightened. There was a sense of 'nothing daunts me.' I noticed that my voice is now stronger in contrast to my usual timid self. Now I am straightforward instead of avoiding issues. Also, I felt taller!"   —NL, London, England

"My husband is a different man on Coconut. He is really dealing with his issues—and he's open to taking his drops."

—GR, Medford, OR

74

"Our humanity were a poor thing were it not for the divinity which stirs within us." —Bacon

FLOWER/FRUIT/FOLKLORE

So named because the ripe coconut resembles a monkey's head, the coconut palm probably originated in the Malay Archipelago over three thousand years ago and now grows along the seashore of many tropical lands. Reaching a height of up to eighty feet, it bears fruit for as many years. Coconut palms are cross-fertilized, as the tiny white male and female flowers do not mature at the same time. The coconut is a large, one-seeded fruit, its fibrous husk enclosing the brown, hard-shelled nut. Coconut milk, made by liquefying the meat, is seventy percent fat, and rich in phosphorus and iron. Comparable to mother's milk in its chemical balance, it is a complete protein food. The milk may be used to treat cataracts and fungal infections.

Quality: Uplifted Spiritual Awareness
Message of Self-mastery: Superconsciousness; endurance; perseverance; for completing tasks; living one's highest potential; strong, steady energy; welcoming challenges; solution-orientation; for readiness to take the next step; determination despite setbacks.
Pattern of Disharmony: For making excuses; lack of endurance; problem-orientation; shakiness; escapism; a quitter; avoidance attitude; for the "last straw" feeling; for the inability to commit to putting out more energy.

SPECTRUM PLACEMENT

Coconut, placed in Quadrant I's second house, is the natural successor to Lettuce. Through Lettuce, we enjoy a clean-slated mind, freed from restlessness and upsetting emotions. Now we take the mind to its highest expression—the superconscious, meaning "above the conscious mind." Problems exist on the conscious level; their solutions, on the superconscious. Coconut embraces both the milky softness of the Spectrum's feminine half and the first Quadrant's freshness.

POSITIVE APPLICATIONS

About twenty years are required for the coconut palm tree to reach a state of full bearing—a perfect symbol for Coconut essence's quality of perseverance. "Patience, endurance attaineth to all," promised the Spanish saint Teresa of Avila. Coconut, then, helps us to commit to resolutions and solutions—and to believe that they are here to be found.

The positive Coconut state is splendid for completing tasks. We live in an age when one's word means so little. We make promises and then break them. We start projects and then quit. In a recent Broadway play, the female lead confessed to her friend that she had once been married. "How long?" he asked. "Oh, I don't know," she replied, "but it seemed like *weeks*." Of course this is a joke, although a sad one, revealing a certain lack of commitment and the express need for the essence of Coconut.

Coconut gives a clearer, more spiritual focus. It will help to give you the energy to endure, or to rise above, every test. It shows us the value of seeing a challenge through to its conclusion, no matter how difficult it is. Poet Robert Frost put it well: "The best way out is always through."

Some years ago, I had the opportunity to personally research Coconut while sitting in the dentist's chair awaiting an impending root canal treatment. Having had one before, I knew I was in for a rough time, being a painful experience at best with an uncomfortable week or so of healing afterward. Beads of sweat gathered profusely on my upper lip in memory of a previous dental visit. "I can just walk out of here right now," came the joyful, albeit cowardly, thought. But no—I was trapped. There was clearly no way out of this test except through what a friend once called "the icky middle."

Then I remembered the bottle of Coconut in my purse and slipped a drop under my tongue. My state of mind changed instantly. Yes, the fear was still there, and so was I. But a subtle change had occurred, thanks to Coconut; I was then able to "get a grip on myself." It was as though I had taken myself by the shoulders and said, "Look, you're just going to have to go through with this. You know from past experience that it will probably hurt, but the good news is, it's going to end."

Coconut is the answer to our shakiness and lack of commitment. This remedy is epitomized by the intestinal fortitude of Olympic competitors who demonstrate superhuman skill and talent, and the ability to pick themselves up when they fall and "try, try again."

"It's not just athletic skill that molds winners," writes John Anderson in an article entitled, "What Makes Olympic Champions?" [9] Answering his own question, Mr. Anderson pinpoints several necessary qualities: having a dream; being fired up; mustering the ability to bounce back; aiming high; having a back-up plan for trouble; never quitting despite setbacks; and making their own luck. In a nutshell, these are all outstanding qualities of Coconut.

Olympic winners, he observed, "mounted the winners' stand not simply because of athletic talent but because of resolute inner fiber. Real winners in sports, as in business or school, are those whose failures inspire them to go at it again. Hanging in there despite setbacks teaches us the value of perseverance. An inner dynamo keeps Olympic champions going—for the possibility of a medal as well as the satisfaction of completing a difficult task against immense odds. That same effort can apply whether the task is a race, a difficult mathematics lesson or a corporate report.

These words of inspiration from 1994 Olympic competitors summarize the positive Coconut state:

"Of course there is a lot of pressure on us in Norway, but that only makes me stronger."   —Espen Bredesen, Norwegian ski jumper
"This time, it's something I can do, not something I have to do. But it's just my nature to go for the gold."   —Cathy Turner, USA speed skater

If we look symbolically at the coconut—the hard shell representing the body, the meaty pulp the mind, and the subtly sweet milk the soul—we find a perfect metaphor for the vibrational message of the positive Coconut state: integration. "A tough nut to crack," Coconut rewards our efforts with superconsciousness.

NEGATIVE INDICATIONS

The defeatist attitude paraphrases a major negative Coconut trait. Coconut's solution is, simply, not to give up. This essence addresses neither Strawberry's self-doubt nor Pineapple's lack of confidence, but rather a mere lack of committed energy. The conscious decision simply to give up or, worse yet never to begin, portrays the negative Coconut state. As W.C. Fields said, comically, "If at first you don't succeed try, try again. Then quit. No use being a damn fool about it." This attitude is an unmistakable cry for Coconut!

The negative Coconut state manifests as procrastination, making excuses, unwillingness, or any form of escapism to avoid getting the job done. "My husband had put off repairing our furniture for so long—a year or more—that I finally gave up on him," wrote Darlene. "Then I remembered Coconut. You should see our living room now! I'm proud to show it off to anyone who visits."

Coconut tells us that every question has an answer, every problem a solution, and every rainbow a pot of gold. But what we do not discover until reading the fine print is that the gold is not as easily attained as we might think—it's more like winning the lottery! A "happily ever after" state of mind has nothing in common with outer realities. Rather, it refers to that "pearl of great price," the inner Coconut state of self-transformation.

THEME CHARACTERISTICS

When confronting challenges, Coconut themes are individuals of great patience and endurance. They will hold a job for many years even under the most adverse circumstances, such as: no heartfelt interest in the work, difficult co-workers or employer/employees, unsatisfactory income, or unhappy working conditions. They are inspirational companions for this very attitude of commitment to seeing a job through to completion. We could say, "they resolve to solve."

Coconut themes are more than born optimists. Their very cells are committed to higher truths. Intuitively, they know that solutions to seemingly unsolvable problems abound. This inner knowing forms the underlying reason for their astounding perseverance.

One characteristic physical attribute of Coconut themes is a strong bone structure, regardless of body weight. Mentally, the quality of stamina is predominant. The magnetism they offer to others is a blending of the qualities of upliftment and perseverance, quietly encouraging us: "If I can do it, so can you."

FAMOUS THEME PERSONALITIES

Arthur Ashe
Cathy Turner
Espen Bredesen
Jacques Cousteau
The Ever-Ready Battery Bunny
Larry Bird
Ludwig van Beethoven
Marcus Tullius
Cicero
Sri Ramakrishna
Plotinus

As a stunning Coconut theme example, Arthur Ashe comes to mind. That he was a champion black tennis player—the first Wimbledon had ever known—almost pales beside his other accomplishments. He also championed justice for blacks, actively opposing South Africa's apartheid. In the early 1990s, he took part in a demonstration protesting the government's treatment of Haitian political refugees. Mr. Ashe epitomized Coconut's ability to persevere in his crusade to eradicate the psychological remnants of slavery. For although slavery officially ended a long time ago, he recognized that racial prejudice has lingered to this day.

Perhaps his greatest test—and the test of his greatness—was his choice to go public with news of the AIDS virus that he had contracted from a blood transfusion during heart surgery in 1983. Mr. Ashe epitomized Coconut's strengths, both in his struggle with AIDS and with his opponents on the tennis courts. Never did he ask, "Why me?" The obstacles on the tennis court and the ravages of AIDS were the same to him, as Coconut-like opportunities for spiritual growth. Arthur Ashe, a champion in every sense of the word, uplifted family, friends, and countless fans through the inspiration of his life as well as his passing. He died in 1993 in his forties.

CONFESSIONS OF A COCONUT THEME: LORENA'S STORY

"I had a very colorful childhood, truthfully, and have thought a lot about writing it. My parents were already separated by the time I was born. They divorced when I was two, and I didn't meet my dad till I was twenty-five. That was pretty interesting, and it was wonderful when I got to meet him. My mom was married three times. I had a family that was very artistic. From a very early age, I was exposed to the arts and absorbed them on a daily basis. That's probably why I became a musician and a violin teacher.

"My mother's life was in such turmoil—she was an alcoholic—that I spent a lot of my childhood alone, parenting myself and taking care of myself physically and emotionally. I've learned to have an enormous amount of persistence in terms of my own emotional healing. I've worked doggedly on that from my earliest memories, really, to find a better way and not be done in by that stuff. It's been a big mountain to climb, but I feel richly rewarded.

"In some ways, yes, I think I have long-haul stamina. I'm a good long-distance runner, but I'm not real fast. I can run and not feel too winded. This kind of sums up my energy. I do have trouble, though, getting bottomed out during the day. But with some time to myself and some sleep, I can just get back up and go.

"I would say that I'm an uplifting person, and I look for this quality in others. I give a lot of support and positive feedback to people in my life, and definitely to my students and the people that I work with. I feel like I'm here to be a vehicle to uplift others.

"I've never been crazy about coconuts. I've not ever developed a relationship with them. But macaroons are good! The other day, my girlfriend gave me some coconut lip gloss and I really liked it."

WRAPPING IT UP

There is a folk saying that he who plants a coconut tree plants vessels and clothing, food and drink, a habitation for himself, and a heritage for his children. What other delicacy from the plant kingdom can make such claims? Likewise, the quality of upliftment, proffered through the tiny coconut flower, is equally all-encompassing. The coconut, growing as high as eighty feet above ground, is itself a symbol of elevated, uplifting qualities. Coconut essence, then, offers us a path out of suffering and into joy. It accompanies us through the dark forest of trials into the light of freedom.

Coconut gives us a fine example of a strong, steady energy. It vibrationally speaks of living fully in the moment, being willing to take risks, and doing what we know to be the right thing, whether it "feels" good or not. The reward for our "stick-to-it-iveness" is upliftment in which, through our efforts, we are raised to a higher level of awareness. Coconut's message is to honor that "divinity which stirs within us."

COCONUT	Contrasted With:	Companioned With:
Corn	for beginning new endeavors rather than sustaining or finishing them	for the energy to initiate and complete undertakings
Orange	perseverance, specifically through periods of depression	to overcome tests that are especially heavy or emotionally trying
Pear	balance in emergencies or related to specific short-term tests	perseverance through especially difficult tests, including emergencies
Tomato	for battling fears or addictions	for longstanding tests with no end in sight where the attitude of a long-distance runner is required

POSITIVE EXPRESSIONS

Expansive

Greater awareness

Completing tasks

Honoring vows

Welcoming challenges

Willing

Realistic

Persevering

Stamina-filled

Patient

Uplifting

Steady

Steadfast

Solution-oriented

Determined

Sense of readiness

Committed

Ready to face difficulties

NEGATIVE CONDITIONS

Defeatist attitude

Low energy-prone

Procrastinating

Finding excuses

Unwilling

Escapist attitude

Problem-oriented

Shaky

Noncommittal

Trapped in the conscious mind

Cowardly

ESSENCE ENHANCERS

Take up a new sport or hobby that stretches you, either physically or mentally, beyond your limits.

Analyze your present life. In one column, list problems—in the other, the solutions. Reflect on both columns, and make needed changes for improvement.

One by one, finish projects that you have left incomplete.

Mentally repeat the Coconut affirmation several times a day, especially when taking this essence.

VISUALIZATION

You have just stepped out onto the ice for one last practice session before the skating competition. How many of those about to watch you realize the intense years of training that have gone into these mere four minutes of performance time? And who among them has experienced your love of skating—the unparalleled freedom of speed and strength on the ice, or the sense of flying with perfect physical control?

The music begins, and you give yourself to it. Gone now are the hours and years of training. Gone now is also the driving desire to win. Only you and the ice exist, connected through the music. "The Blue Danube" blares through the loudspeakers, though to you, it seems to rise up out of the ice beneath your skates. All you need to do is give yourself to the music.

Using your arms and legs to pick up speed, you jump and spin. The familiar breeze through your hair and the coldness on your ears spur you on. Skating is always the same—so freeing, so empowering. Again, you jump, pushing up out of the ice, as it were, to lift yourself up and out of it. All the dance, gymnastics, and yoga postures have made these moments possible. All the fluidity and sense of rhythm are yours, through countless hours of discipline.

Music becomes movement, and movement becomes grace. Now, at last, you are ready for the performance.

AFFIRMATION:

I see every obstacle as an opportunity to rise in inner happiness and freedom!

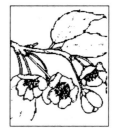

Prunus avium
("sweet plum of the birds")

CHAPTER TWELVE

CHERRY:
"THE GOOD CHEER
MESSENGER"

"I put my husband on Cherry. Now he is acting differently. He is more relaxed, and smiles more often. He made dinner for us last week, and even enjoyed cooking it."
                                                    —RJ, Evanston, IL

"My wife took Cherry, and was whistling away!"
                                                    — TM, Ontario, Canada

"I felt an upbeat energy from Cherry—cheerful, actually."
                                                    —RL, Denton, TX

"It's almost an instantaneous thing (results from Cherry). It's much like a heavy veil lifting off. "
                                                    —SR, Boise, ID

"I had a client who sobbed uncontrollably during a massage. I felt that she was not cleansing but rather was overwrought. I put two drops of Cherry in her massage oil and she stopped immediately."
                                                    —NB, Nevada City, CA

"Even as we spoke over the phone and you suggested Cherry, I felt a great joy. When you're pregnant, you feel so unlike yourself! I felt better and had more energy while taking it."   —MB, Tempe AZ

"You cannot prevent the birds of sorrow from flying over your head, but you can prevent them from building nests in your hair."—Chinese proverb

FLOWER/FRUIT/FOLKLORE

Cherry trees are either sweet or sour. Sweet cherry trees are sensitive and need plenty of space around them to ensure enough sunlight to ripen the fruit. The sour variety, *prunus cerasus,* is among the hardiest of all fruit trees—resistant to harsh weather, insects, and disease. The sweet cherry most likely originated in Asia Minor, its many varieties dating back to Roman times. In fact, cherry pits have been found in prehistoric cave dwellings. The trees' white or pinkish flowers grow in clusters on long stalks or pedicels, producing the shiny fruit with a single stone. Cherries are high in iron, act as a laxative and a blood builder, rid the body of toxins, and stimulate the glandular system. The juice is an excellent tonic for gout and hacking coughs. One of its lesser known usages is as a remedy to counteract food poisoning from fish.

Quality: Cheerfulness
Message of Self-mastery: Light-hearted; hope; inspiration to others; seeing the good in everything; optimistic; positive; the ability to make light of difficulties; genuine, soul-stirring laughter; even-mindedness.
Pattern of Disharmony: Moodiness; grumpiness; fault-finding; "waking up on the wrong side of the bed"; contrariness; ornery; feeling mildly to moderately emotionally out of control; moods of known and unknown origin; for the need to "snap out of it."

SPECTRUM PLACEMENT

Cherry finds its placement midway through Quadrant I's third house. At this halfway point, we see the quality of lightness at its peak in Cherry's carefree spirit. From Coconut's message of upliftment and a growing commitment to carve our own lives, Cherry emerges. Its childlike first-Quadrant buoyancy with a delicate femininity is a necessary building block in creating a happy sense of self.

POSITIVE APPLICATIONS

Symbolic of Cherry's ability to help dispel surface-layer moods, the cherry tree itself is shallow-rooted—less than two feet underground. Much like the human temperament, it produces fruit that is either sweet or sour.

Cherry sports a bubbly quality reminiscent of children's songs and stories: Mary Poppins singing, "Just a Spoonful of Sugar Helps the Medicine Go Down"; "Whistle While You Work" from Cinderella; and of course, the seven dwarfs singing, "Hi ho, hi ho, it's off to work we go." Are these songs pure fiction and fantasy? Let's hope not! We adults have a lot to learn from their simple wisdom. The old folk saying that "life is like a bowl of cherries" can apply to every one of us with a simple change of attitude.

In the positive Cherry state, we are able to see the good in people and things. We smile more. We skip in step a bit. We resonate with the bumper sticker message that reminds us, "Don't worry, be happy." Without moods clouding the mind, emotional steadiness is our natural state.

Another important characteristic of Cherry is the refreshing quality of even-mindedness, and with it, a certain detachment. Emotional investment in the outcome of life's tests is equivalent to asking for a mood. And don't we all, even consciously at times, choose to court them? Referring to Coconut's lottery metaphor, why be distraught if you don't win? One in the positive Cherry state is a good loser; healthy indifference is his victory.

NEGATIVE INDICATIONS

The negative Cherry state reflects our decision to be negative, pessimistic, or just plain unhappy. Molehills become mountains and small chores turn into large burdens. It seems there is no right side of the bed on which to wake up! Thus, we see the tongue-in-cheek definition of a pessimist as "someone who complains about the noise when opportunity knocks." Those in the negative Cherry state view life as a disappointment waiting to happen—which it invariably does, just as they predicted.

To put the matter directly—if you make up your mind to be happy, nothing in the world can make you unhappy. Conversely, if you decide to be unhappy, nothing can cheer you. It seems self-evident here that the main issue is choice. At any given moment, we are making choices in our lives. Granted, we cannot control the events that befall us, such as the birds of sorrow flying overhead. But we can control how we react to them by choosing not to invite them to nest in our hair!

Caught in the negative Cherry state, the legendary film star Katherine Hepburn once said, "I don't know what one means by 'happy.' I'm happy spasmodically. If I eat a chocolate Turtle, I'm happy. When the box is empty, I'm unhappy. When I get another box, I'm happy again." Tell me—do any of us truly covet a state of happiness so fragile that it can come and go on mere whim?

When we invite the negative Cherry state into our minds, before long we find ourselves in a mood that begins to snowball. In time, tracing this emotional blemish back to its point of origin is difficult at best. All we know is that we're not happy. At this point, the mood takes control of us and everything look bleak. We tend to view the world, innocuous though it may be, from our own state of consciousness. "Wind on a hill sounds lonely if you're sad," writes J. Donald Walters, "free if you're free, cheerful if you're glad."

THEME CHARACTERISTICS

A vibrant cheeriness is the hallmark of the Cherry theme. Here we find someone who often, though not always, has suffered through a difficult childhood and emerged without emotional scarring. His good nature cannot be marred by a family history of substance abuse, debilitating bouts of physical illness, divorce, or even several unhappy marriages.

Cherry themes seem untouched by the dream nature of this world. Their earlier years, like moods or bad dreams, evaporate as though they had never happened. These people have a distinctive lightness of step and a buoyancy to their gait. Often, though not always, they are rosy-cheeked, similar to Raspberry themes. The optimism of the Cherry state is contagious "in a most delightful way," to quote Mary Poppins. Cherry themes cheer us. They make us laugh.

FAMOUS THEME PERSONALITIES

Mary Poppins

Shirley Temple Black

Goldie Hawn

Johnny Carson

Happy (of the seven dwarfs)

Benjamin Franklin

Soupy Sales

Kathy Najimy

Ellen DeGeneres

Whoopi Goldberg

Mary Poppins is, for all children and all time, the legendary nanny who blows in on the east wind. You will find her caretaking, and routinely astounding, the Banks children who reside at Number Seventeen on—coincidentally—Cherry-Tree Lane. Although seemingly of a sour and no-nonsense of disposition, Ms. Poppins evokes the most delightful cheerfulness in all who know her. She turns medicine into lime juice cordial and life into a carnival. She will remain in children's hearts long after the shifting winds have whisked her away.

The Mary Poppins of literature is portrayed a great deal more stiffly than the Poppins of film. The literary version, prim and proper, suggests a strong Fig sub-theme, adding an element of paradox to her character. Ms. Poppins, who just "popped in," is actually more complex than she seems, for this very Fig-like reason. We might be tempted to label her a Fig theme with a Cherry sub-theme, except for one give-away clue—the pervasive, childlike joy that her magnetism evokes in others. (Remember to look for "magnetism clues"—or how your subject's energy affects others around him—in assessing themes.) Do as you're told, Poppins energetically commands, and we'll make it more fun than you could ever imagine.

CONFESSIONS OF A CHERRY THEME: LISA'S TALE

"I would say that my biggest quirk is that, even though I do psychic readings for people and have the ability to be very compassionate, I also really tend to laugh at people's foibles. When I start doing the readings, I start to chuckle, sometimes when people are almost in tears. But I think it's because life is ridiculous in a way, and so absurd. It's hard to see it when we're the ones going through problems. But I do find some stuff very funny.

"I had a pretty bleak childhood in many ways. I grew up in a big family. I think I was very lonely, even though there were a lot of kids around. My father was very abusive, and that was hard for me. School was incredibly boring, but I felt safe there, so it was okay. As soon as I could, I moved away. I felt, 'If I don't get away from here, I'm going to die.' There was a really strong sense of spiritual death—so lonely, nobody with the same kind of values. But it taught me a lot about programming and how the brain works, and how important it is to overcome our past experiences to a degree.

"I deal with my emotions intellectually, but I do deal with them. For three years I've been in hormonal turmoil—being pregnant, nursing, and then starting with hot flashes and what not. I've been told that with me, what you see is what you get. If I'm upset you can see it all over my face. If I'm sad or touched, I just cry. When I'm happy, it's just right there. I don't repress things very well.

"I don't see how people survive without a sense of humor. I can't see any reason to at least not continually take anything in this world seriously. Laughing, I think, frees our energy to move forward and to not be limited by this physical plane. The quality that made me just certain that my marriage would work was that my husband could make me laugh and just have a sense of humor regardless of whatever might be happening. We can pretty much get a chuckle out of almost anything. That was incredibly important to me. And it's helped me often. (chuckle)

"Oh, I love cherries. I could eat cherries all day and all night. And I wish I could!"

WRAPPING IT UP

Some years ago, I was fortunate to spend a vacation secluding at a friend's oceanside cabin. The rustic stonework and wood and the absence of electricity and phone all contributed to the perfect hideaway that I had been craving. The only flaw was my growing attitude of attachment to the place. My lesson was to learn that if we find joy within ourselves, we needn't look for it elsewhere.

I would soon be leaving, I thought, and my good cheer became tinged with gloom. With great reluctance, I packed up and prepared to leave. And then came the hitch—my car wouldn't start. I was stranded in a prison that only moments before had seemed a paradise! Clearly, the cabin had not changed. Unbeknownst to me, I had simply entered the negative Cherry state.

The moral of this story is that circumstances are always neutral. This truth was known to Benjamin Franklin who wisely said of material possessions, "Money never made a man happy yet, nor will it. There is nothing in its nature to produce happiness."

The message of Cherry, then, is about having a more lighthearted, less heavy attitude toward life. Life is what we make of it. And herein lies the greatest hope. We have heard the saying that one man's tea is another man's poison. The drink in question either delights or destroys us according to our own perception of it, not the actual contents. Cherry, in its unique, light-hearted way, helps us with that decision. "What, me mope? Nope!" is this essence's motto.

CHERRY	Contrasted With:	Companioned With:
Blackberry	for negativity due to a critical nature rather than moods	for pure happiness
Grape	for the ability to "see the larger reality" with equanimity	for a playful, loving nature; finding fulfillment within ourselves
Orange	for deep-rooted depression and an inability to lift oneself out of it	for an energetic understanding that joy on all levels is our true nature
Raspberry	for kindheartedness in relation to others and not only oneself	to balance lightness with depth of insight and empathy
Spinach	for lightheartedness born of trust and the simple nature of a child	to awaken our developmentally nourished childlike spirit

POSITIVE EXPRESSIONS

Light-hearted	Even-minded
Childlike	Optimistic
Cheerful	Positive
Bubbly	Emotionally stable
Light-spirited	Untouched by difficulties
Happy	Contented
Spontaneous	

NEGATIVE CONDITIONS

Negative	Determined to remain upset
Pessimistic	Caught in a "dark cloud"
Unhappy	Brooding
Sad	Temperamental
Self-pitying	Heavy-spirited
Gloomy	Grumpy
Moody	Of sour disposition

ESSENCE ENHANCERS

Spend time with children Try to understand their reality through shared activities.

Nip moods in the bud. If you can't change them immediately, change your environment. Go out for a walk, a meal, or a movie.

Read fairy tales or stories of heroes and heroines to children.

Sing, dance or be a little bit silly.

Whistle, or learn to.

VISUALIZATION

Sit back and close your eyes. When you open them, imagine yourself sitting in the middle of a cherry tree orchard, right in the middle of the biggest tree that is ripe with cherries. Still young enough to count your age on the fingers of one hand, you study your tiny, cherry-stained appendages, pleased with yourself that you know how to count.

Yes, you snuck away again to have your fill of the sweet fruit—and who could blame you? Without anyone having to say anything, you know you are eating the light-hearted playfulness of the cherries—and that is what makes them so sweet.

A gentle breeze roves through the orchard, filling your nostrils with the flowery scent. A maverick cloud sneaks across the sky, as afraid to be caught as you are, doing something it was told not to do. Surrounded by branches dripping cherry clusters and so many feet above the ground, life seems just a touch unreal. From this height, it is easy to be detached. From this sense of detachment a pleasant cheerfulness, like the scent of sweet cherries, wafts upward to the treetops.

Into this gentle breeze, let your cares dissolve. Watch all your worries and moods fly away. And let that very sweet, soft joy become a twinkle in your eye.

AFFIRMATION

I swim gaily on the sea of life, joyfully breasting the dancing waves of bliss!

CHAPTER THIRTEEN

SPINACH:

"THE UNCOMPLICATOR"

Spinacea oleracea
("aromatic, prickly-seeded
sweet herb")

"On the second or third day of Spinach, it seemed that my attitude had relaxed and become a little more playful. Because I currently have a high-pressure job as an aerospace engineer and am in the process of a divorce, Spinach helps me with childlike qualities."

—*JN, Mountain View, CA*

"I love Spinach and feel it may be my theme essence. Just after taking it, I felt very meditative, then spacey, and then euphoric."

—*JS, North San Juan, CA*

"I took Spinach to help me deal with the death of a close loved one. I felt stressed, on edge, emotional, depressed. On the second day, I experienced an increase in creativity, healing dreams, and a comical perspective on the situation."

—*MG, Palo Alto, CA*

"I gave Spinach to one of my clients—a skeptic. She confided that she woke up the next morning 'feeling like a little kid.'"

—*JS, Sacramento, CA*

"When I take Spinach, I remember the things I did as a child that brought me joy. My husband commented, 'Why, you're just like a little child.'"

—*LD, Salt Lake City, UT*

"The child is father of the man." —Wordsworth

FLOWER/FRUIT/FOLKLORE

History records the origin of spinach as Iran and neighboring countries. This vegetable made its way to America in the 1800's. Spinach is a quick-growing potherb. A leafy green plant grown solely for its foliage, it is an annual of the goosefoot family, because its leaves are shaped like goose feet. Small, yellowish-white female flowers grow in auxiliary clusters once the plant bolts, its green male flowers growing on the two-foot-high leafy stem. Spinach is especially rich in vitamins A, C, and iron. As a dark green, leafy vegetable, it inhibits cancerous cell mutation and its manganese content is helpful for diabetes. Abundant in therapeutic value, spinach strengthens the lymphatic, urinary, intestinal, and digestive systems.

Qualities: Simplicity, Guilelessness
Message of Self-mastery: Childlike zeal; without guile; trust; sense of wonder, awe, playfulness; freedom; adventurousness; carefree nature.
Pattern of Disharmony: Stress; feeling burdened or overwhelmed; mild distrust to paranoia; for an unhappy or dysfunctional childhood; "worry wart."

SPECTRUM PLACEMENT

Placed in Quadrant I's fourth house, Spinach bespeaks both simplicity and playfulness. Spinach captures Cherry's joy and adds its own two cents' worth of delight. Whereas Cherry symbolizes song and dance, Spinach represents fun and games. This vegetable, made famous by Popeye the Sailor Man, vibrationally allows the child within us to come out and play.

Although the first-Quadrant essences are both childlike and "springish"—the lighter side of the Spectrum—Spinach sports no lack of depth or importance in the grander Spectrum scheme. It's gentle, feminine nature expresses a profound receptivity to life. Spinach lays the necessary groundwork for the loved child to mature into the loving adult. Fun-seeking Spinach is aptly placed in this Quadrant; it is the necessary precursor to Peach.

POSITIVE APPLICATIONS

There is a saying that angels fly because they take themselves lightly. This also describes being in the positive Spinach state. Carefree but not careless, light-footed but not light-headed, Spinach is the child of our Spectrum. The jokester, the punster, the incorrigible humorist—Spinach, similar to Cherry, makes us laugh. Laughter being the best medicine, as authorities tell us, did you know that one hundred belly-aching, side-splitting laughs provide the aerobic equivalent of ten minutes of rowing? That's one way to get yourself in shape!

All of us can benefit from Spinach at one time or another in our lives. It's the great lightener of burdens. Spinach integrates a sense of play with responsibility and wonderment with acceptance. To understand this essence more fully, watch children at play. In the positive Spinach state, life is a game—and that game is pure fun.

For indications of the presence of Spinach qualities, look into children's eyes. Even the eyes of baby animals reflect that sense of innocence, trust, and play. We might in fact call a baby elephant—our weight many times over—"cute." People in the positive Spinach state are like children. They relate to their environment, including their own bodies, with an attitude of, "Wow, this is really something! Let's see what I can do with it."

NEGATIVE INDICATIONS

As Lord Byron lyricized in the early 1800's, "Ah! happy years! Once more who would not be a boy!" To answer his rhetorical question— the individual manifesting the negative Spinach state. The glories of youth as portrayed by many a poet are considered undesirable to those in the negative Spinach state. These poor souls, alas, are too busy, too important, or too worried to pay attention to the precious life stage of childhood.

One of the sad "occupational hazards" of the work environment in today's world is stress. The dictionary defines stress as "strain or pressure, especially a force that strains or deforms." The psychological deformities caused by stress, such as worry and nervousness, can feed chemical poisons into our bodies, triggered by the brain. Warning signs in the physical body—such as headaches, indigestion, high blood pressure, and knotted shoulder muscles—mean it is time for Spinach. To remain free of "worldly wisdom" and pretentiousness, this essence of guilelessness is paramount.

At the end of the first day of a holistic trade show several years ago, a woman came to our booth with a splitting headache caused by the visual overload customary to these events. We shared a few words, and then I mentioned Spinach—not for the headache, but for feeling overwhelmed and sensorily bombarded. (As previously explained, flower remedies do not directly address physical symptoms.) She returned the next day with one of the most frequent responses to the essences, saying, "After taking Spinach, I felt like myself again." She explained how she had decided to walk to the auditorium that morning instead of driving. As she approached the metal spikes at the parking lot exit point with the warning sign, "Do not back up: severe tire damage," she thought, "I wonder what those feel like"—and then gently stepped on them, out of sheer curiosity. It was a very "Spinach" thing to do!

Much attention is being given these days to the concept of the inner child and the quality of the childhood that we experienced. If it was dysfunctional—meaning that our psycho-physiological needs were not met and nurtured in a healthy way—how then can we grow into functional adults and be expected to carry on normal, healthy relationships? Spinach addresses these unmet needs from childhood that, sooner or later, can manifest as dysfunction.

THEME CHARACTERISTICS

The Spinach theme is truly fun-loving. Easily spotted by a playfulness in the eyes and a contagious, slightly impish smile, this theme is overtly childlike—and sometimes a prankster or slapstick comedian as well! He tends to draw out the child in others and will make friends readily. Several summers ago, I attended a picnic with a Spinach theme girlfriend. Although in her early forties, she had found her way into a watermelon seed-spitting contest with a group of children. The other kids didn't stand a chance of beating her.

Spinach themes enjoy role-playing and dressing up. Similar to Cherry themes, they like to tickle our psyches. Their humor is delightful, though, to be honest, not always profound. And they are usually the first to laugh at their own jokes—that by the way, are not always funny. Their gait has a weightless quality no matter what their age. Their bodies, even if older, retain a youthful air. Spinach themes relish the simple things in life, shying away from extravagant tastes while possessing a boundless ability for enjoyment. In their presence, you will feel delightfully refreshed—and notably younger!

FAMOUS THEME PERSONALITIES
Winnie The Pooh
Robin Williams
P. G. Wodehouse
Kevin Kline
Peter Pan
Tom Sawyer
Ed Wynn
Laurel & Hardy
Victor Borge
The Three Stooges

Who but Edward the Bear, a.k.a., Winnie-the-Pooh, can we profile as our idyllic Spinach theme? None other than Christopher Robin's fuzzy friend who believes that honey was created for one purpose only—him! Pooh personifies the simplicity of Spinach at its most charming expression possible. "Let's go and see *everybody*," he says. "Because when you've been walking in the wind for miles, and you suddenly go into somebody's house, and he says, 'Hallo, Pooh, you're just in time for a little smackerel of something,' and you are, then it's what I call a friendly day."

In this story the innocent Pooh goes to visit his friend, Owl, just to wish him a Happy Thursday—a perfect "Spinach" greeting. Being a blusterous day in the Hundred Acre Wood, his companion Piglet worries that a tree might fall on them. Pooh responds with flawless, Spinach-like trust, "Supposing it didn't." His reply reveals the uncomplicated mind of a true Spinach theme—too simple to even warrant a sub-theme!

CONFESSIONS OF A SPINACH THEME: IN RHODA'S WORDS

"Any quirks? Well, this is probably just my love of fun and the whimsical. I see things in a different light than most people. I mean, I go to the grocery store and I look at how the vegetables are shaped, you know, and I see little stories happening. So I keep myself very entertained and amused. But I enjoy beautiful things, and I'm very visual. I just kind of see the world that way. I have fun. I think you have to take yourself lightly for all the other stuff that comes your way. If you don't take yourself too seriously, then you can handle the traumas that happen to you in a lighter vein.

"I had a very nice childhood with two very loving parents. I had a wonderful time—a very good school experience and lots of really good friends. You hate to say it was an Ozzie-and-Harriet life, but it pretty much was. I grew up in the 1950's. It was a good time to grow up, before the drugs and all the heavy-duty stuff started. I was brought up to be very responsible. And even though that's good, it can hang you up as much as being a 'flake' all your life.

"I would say that I'm a trusting person. And I stay away from stress by not putting limits on myself. One can do so much without setting limits. I've watched people come into the store to work and get stressed out. They say, 'Gosh, I'm really tired today, or 'I can't do this today.' And I would see that pretty soon they don't have any energy! Mentally, we sabotage our own energy. And it's a socially acceptable thing to do. It's so easy to complain, 'Oh, yes, I've worked so hard.' I think we're really not as busy as we think we are. It's just a matter, really, of where we put our priorities.

"Oh, yes, I do like spinach — as long as it's not canned. I seek it out occasionally. We even grew spinach in our garden at one time. It's a nice, leafy vegetable—good color, good shape."

WRAPPING IT UP

Spinach is a plain and uncomplicated plant, ready for the table in a mere forty days. It grows in cool weather. Yet for all its simplicity, Spinach offers a wealth of vitamins and minerals. In addition to its rich physical nourishment is its abundance of essence qualities. Its depth lies in its awareness of the importance of taking ourselves lightly, living without guile, and enjoying all the seasons of our lives.

"Call not that man wretched, who whatever ills he suffers, has a child to love," wrote the poet Southey. If that child resides comfortably within us, so much the better. Spinach, then, could be described as "bottled childhood." It offers us the opportunity to recapture our youth and to rejoice in the delicate play of life. Spinach profiles a consciousness of simplicity through the child emerging, and the child fully healed.

SPINACH	Contrasted With:	Companioned with:
Almond	for stress due to over-extending one's energy	for a tension-free, fun-loving attitude
Cherry	cheerfulness from the absence of moods and cloudy emotions	to awaken our developmentally nourished childlike spirit
Orange	for an abusive childhood	to vibrationally remove the residual effects of a dysfunctional childhood
Peach	for the unconditionally loving mother	whole parent, whole child, within the same individual

POSITIVE EXPRESSIONS

Simple-natured

Trusting

Buoyant

Respectful of life

Attuned with nature

Appreciative

Enthusiastic

Honest

Innocent

Free-spirited

Exuberant

Desirous of exploring

Curious

Friendly

Interested

Pure

Playful

Without guile or pretension

Sincere

Living within one's means

Satisfied with simple things

Lover of animals

Humorous

Nature loving

NEGATIVE CONDITIONS

Overly intellectual

Discontent

Stress-prone

Afraid of aging

Worrisome

Overwhelmed

Taking oneself too seriously

Overburdened

Overly-analytical

Unhappy childhood roots

Dysfunctional childhood

Mischievous

Shrewd

Humorless

Humorous

Nature loving

ESSENCE ENHANCERS

Play games with children.

Spend time in the sun—with lots of sunscreen!

Visit the zoo or a pet store.

Go camping or backpacking.

Go to places frequented by children—the ice skating rink, roller rink, water slide park, or a children's matinee.

Go to a magic show; ride a hot-air balloon; visit the circus or amusement park.

VISUALIZATION

Sit quietly with closed eyes. Imagine that you are reaching upward, grabbing a pleasant experience from your childhood—much like taking hold of the string of a helium-filled balloon. Whatever the memory, allow the details to drift; hold only to the pleasant remembrance of that memory's spirit. Perhaps you feel a warmth, a sense of security, a calm assuredness that all is right. Whatever that feeling, bathe yourself in it now.

Let the quality of simplicity surround you like a springtime breeze in mid-afternoon. Simple, carefree, trusting: these are the colors of childhood. These are the qualities washing from your thoughts all stress, over-concern, and overwhelm.

Now relax even more deeply. Visualize yourself at the foot of a small forested hill. The sun-cloaked pine branches beckon you to step forward. A few yards ahead, a young speckled fawn dashes onto the footpath, startling both of you. She freezes; you crouch down slowly. The fawn responds to your inner voice that says, "Don't be afraid. I'm as curious as you." Her tiny ears draw back in timid wonder. Too young to know fear and sensing your gentleness, she steps forward and sniffs your outstretched palm. As she does so, you look into her eyes, so new to this world. You see in them the innocent joy of youth and the simple magic of childhood.

Embrace the memory of the fawn's eyes, again like taking hold of a balloon. Remember that you, too, cradle a child inside.

AFFIRMATION

Whatever comes to me is for my highest good! I welcome it!

CHAPTER FOURTEEN

PEACH:
"THE SELFLESS MOTHER"

Prunus persica
("peach plum tree")

"I am a nurse in a small rural East Coast clinic and just started Peach. One night last week, the doctor called. Often when this happens, he asks me to do something that is his responsibility, something I really don't want to do. I tend to shut down to him as a result and don't extend to him the same servicefulness I do to others. This time, though, I answered cheerfully, 'Yes, Doctor, what can I do for you?' being somewhat amazed at my own response. The doctor said that the work had been done, and would I like to come over for brownies!"

—*SP, Bristol, RI*

"I want you to know that I felt the wonderful effect of the Peach drops within a few hours after taking them. I became a different person with much less concern for myself that helped me to focus on so many other things. What a wonderful feeling it gave me!"

—*MR, Scottsdale, AZ*

"I took Peach somewhat reluctantly. I didn't notice changes, but my boss commented that he was more pleased than ever with my work."

—*MC, Boulder, CO*

"On Peach, I noticed that I wrote better letters to my friends and communicated more clearly." —*RH, Santa Fe, NM*

"I took Peach at 730 a.m. two days ago. I felt very accepting. I got on the train to work, sat down beside this person and started talking to him and shared things that were personal to me—this was not like me! Then at work, I called my parents just to say 'hi,' called a business friend I hadn't spoken to in months, and even called my ex-wife! It's like, I really wanted to step into other people's shoes and see how it felt."

—*LK, Seattle, WA*

> *"Men resemble the gods in nothing so much as in doing*
> *good to their fellow creatures."*   —Cicero

FLOWER/FRUIT/FOLKLORE

The peach is 4,000 years old. Its native home is China where it was venerated as a fruit of immortality. In his writings in the fifth century B.C., Confucius refers to the "tao," the Chinese word for peach. The tree—small, deciduous, and short-lived—grows in warm, temperate zones. The blossoms of the peach tree are either small and rose pink, or larger and pale pink. The fruit itself may vary considerably in size and color. Peaches are high in vitamin A and are easily assimilated by the body. They are alkalizing to the blood, stimulating to the digestion, and moisturizing to the skin.

Quality: Unselfishness
Message of Self-mastery: Concern for the welfare of others; empathy; maturity; nurturance; consideration; compassion; sensitivity to the needs of others; giving from wholeness instead of neediness.
Pattern of Disharmony: Selfishness; self-involvement; thoughtlessness; "looking out for Number One"; constrictiveness; exploitive nature; inability to relate to other's realities; a tendency to smother; those who sap the energy of their listener; inability to receive love.

SPECTRUM PLACEMENT

Placed in Quadrant I's fifth and last house, Peach embodies the qualities of wonder, newness, and untiring energy in early bloom. Whereas its Spinach predecessor epitomizes the child whose needs are honored and met, Peach now directs that energy outward from its own sense of wholeness toward nurturing others. It is called the "mothering essence." The Peach mother has a light touch and a refreshing energy, much like a breeze in springtime, characteristic of Quadrant I's youthful qualities. Peach sports no heavy-handedness. Also the last of the feminine essences, it gives birth, in a sense, to the masculine half of the Spectrum and Quadrant II, beginning with Corn.

POSITIVE APPLICATIONS

Expansive love and thinking of other's needs before one's own are the hallmarks of Peach. Here we see the mother who feeds her children before sitting down to eat her own meal. Her nourishment is derived from nurturing others. In the positive Peach state, we discover a love that is given freely without condition and with no strings attached.

Some years ago, a young man we'll call Jon who had recently started a jewelry business, came for a consultation. He explained that he'd been struggling financially and was basically frustrated by the numerous difficulties involved in being self-employed and beginning a business. It seemed that he needed to get more in touch with his true motives for the work that he had chosen, and so I suggested Peach. A week later, Jon called to say that his business had picked up, along with his interest in genuinely serving his customers.

Peach is excellent for teachers of students of all ages, for caregivers of the young, and for mothers. It is also of benefit to people starting out in business, for individuals who are self-employed, and for those in managerial or leadership roles. People in sales professions who are good at their jobs have an abundance of Peach traits. They understand that their success is dependent upon befriending their clients, and holding their best interests in mind and helping to meet their needs.

NEGATIVE INDICATIONS

The negative Peach state expresses itself in an unmagnetic and unpleasant manner. It embodies the qualities of giving with selfish or ulterior motives that pollutes an otherwise pure energy. An individual manifesting negative Peach traits is more concerned with "what's in it for me" than in offering quality work and truly helping others. Self-involvement, egocentrism, and a basically selfish nature are all symptomatic of the negative Peach state. These unflattering qualities repel others. They tend to create a sense of loneliness through the inability to cultivate enduring and endearing friendships.

Depression is the fruit of negative Peach's "poor me" attitude. Focusing on the unfulfillment of one's own needs to the exclusion of the larger picture is a guaranteed source of unhappiness. "I was sad that I had no new shoes," the story goes, "until I saw someone without legs."

THEME CHARACTERISTICS

I consulted only yesterday with Tara, a Peach theme. When asked to share any information about herself that she felt was pertinent, she volunteered that raising two children had been an important part of her life and that she had not breast-feed them. "Why did I say *that?*" she later commented. Probably because it was a clue to her theme essence. Tara is a third-grade teacher who pays special attention to creating a warm, nature-filled environment in her classroom. She had chosen to intellectually nurture her students rather than be demonstrative. After her own children left home, she remodeled her bedroom and painted it a pale shade of—what else—peach. Tara loves peaches but, true to the theme characteristic of particularity, only the Freestone variety at their peak of ripeness.

Peach themes are easily spotted by their gentle smiles and a certain fluidity to their gait and movements. Their body language is graceful with a somewhat slow rhythm. Calm and gentle, their energy seems to constantly ask, "What can I do for you?" You may find that you feel accepted, cared for and at ease in their presence. They evoke within us the desire to think of the needs of others before our own.

Peach themes help us to expand our own consciousness. If you find yourself too caught up in your problems, or if life isn't going the way you'd like it to, spend time with a Peach theme. Their company can provide a perspective that your problems are possibly not as looming or lasting as they may seem.

FAMOUS THEME PERSONALITIES

Cinderella
Audrey Hepburn
Mother Teresa of Calcutta
John Denver
Florence Nightingale
Donald Walters
Paul Newman
Sally Struthers
Jimmy Carter

In the realm of best-loved fairy tales, Cinderella exemplifies the perfect Peach theme. This gentle-spirited woman possesses an inner beauty born of selfless loving that remains unmarred by the hearth ashes in which she is forced to sleep—thus her name, Cinder-ella. She also emanates the Peach theme's ability to commune with nature, evoking a response from animals and plants alike. In the original version of this fairy tale as told by the Brothers Grimm, it is "white pigeons, doves, and all the birds under heaven" who help Cinderella complete her stepmother's endless tasks designed to keep her from the prince's ball. And it's not a fairy godmother, but a white bird who creates her magnificent wardrobe for the gala event.

Giving equal love and selfless service to both her pet mice and cruel step-family, it is easy to understand her just reward in the form of the charming prince. (Plus, she got a great pair of dress shoes.) The moral of the story: if we give love, that love is magnetically drawn to us in return.

We may credit Cinderella with a strong Raspberry sub-theme for not harboring bitter or vengeful thoughts toward those who treated her so poorly. Alas, even fairy tales offer no shelter from the abuse of dysfunctional families! Selflessly loving, with accents of Raspberry's unconditional forgiveness, this make-believe character models for us the most beautiful of human qualities.

Confessions of a Peach Theme: Georgia Speaks

"I never wanted children, not even in the slightest. I never liked playing with dolls—it wasn't part of my thing to do. But I like children a lot, actually. I always had really close friends as a child, and I have a strong loyalty streak.

"I am very concerned for the welfare of other people. *Very.* I think I'm fairly sensitive so that when people hurt, I hurt too. I'd like to be able to alleviate their suffering in whatever way possible. Mostly, it takes the form of counseling, empathizing, and sympathizing. I am mothering. I like to nurture. It's broader, though, like a world nurturer. I just always have this sense that I have so many, many children to help.

"Selflessness is something I'm really working on. I think it's a great idea. And next to my meditation, service is the most important thing in my life.

"I love animals and everything in nature—animals and plants. I particularly love plants. I feel when I'm around plants and animals that they give me back energy, just lots of healing. When I work in my herb garden, the plants talk to me and I talk to them. It's how I am fed. I discovered in life that I'm very much happier if I have an herb garden. It makes me feel safe, grounded, calm. There's a patch in my herb garden where I can go and lay down right in the middle of all of my herbs—a very sweet, pure energy.

"I love peaches. But I never have found peaches to suit me quite as well in California as when we could get Georgia peaches back in Tennessee. My mother used to peel them and feed them to me. They were really juicy. I never have been able to get enough peaches. I just was thinking the other day how sad it is in the winter when you can't get peaches. All you get is apples, bananas, and oranges. Peaches are luscious; peaches are juicy; peaches are pretty."

Wrapping It Up

Certainly we would all agree that we are living in hard times—economically, environmentally, and politically. Clearly, our world is suffering.

More than ever, we see the need for the nurturing love epitomized by the archetypal mother. Isn't it the responsibility of each of us, then, to emulate this quality' "In giving, we receive," echoes the essence of Peach. Through sharing, we become peacemakers.

I am fortunate to live in a spiritual community that, if we were to assess its theme essence, would be Peach. Our country was founded on the noble principals of freedom and equality. Similarly, Ananda World Brotherhood Village is based on the striving for inner freedom. This same spirit fosters an attitude among its residents of willingness to help others. Modeling Peach-like ideals, we share with others the joy that we experience on a daily basis through lives dedicated to compassion, cooperation, and service.

PEACH	Contrasted With:	Companioned With:
Date	for judging others	for sensitivity to others; for sweetening relationships
Grape	for unconditional love	for selfless love, loving service
Raspberry need	for sympathy, forgiveness, not "laying trips" on others	"being there" for those in
Spinach	for the healthy child	for healthy parenting of our children and ourselves
Strawberry	for a healthy self-image	for integrity developed through the act of giving; conscious mothering with healthy boundaries

POSITIVE EXPRESSIONS

Selfless

Genuinely interested in others

Secure in self

Understanding

Sensitive

Good listener

Compassionate

Caring

Nurturing

Altruistic

Humanitarian

Concerned

Generous

Helpful

Unconditionally loving

Does tasks well

Pure

Gentle

Kind

Pure of motives

Supportive

Appreciative

Joyful

NEGATIVE CONDITIONS

Smothering

Self-involved

Self-seeking

Garrulous

Talking about self

Narrow

Martyr state of mind

Lonely

Greedy

Advice-giving, unsolicited

Egocentric

Unable to see the bigger picture

Disinterested in others

Inconsiderate

Insensitive

Rude

Unappreciative

Depressed

"Me first" attitude

Exploitive

Manipulative

Uses guilt

Needy

Feeling inadequate

Domineering

Meddlesome

"Strings attached" attitude

ESSENCE ENHANCERS

Do volunteer work, especially helping those less fortunate than yourself.

Work with children. If you have friends who are single mothers, offer to spend time with their children.

Donate money to worthy causes and tithe on a monthly basis.

Have pets, and learn to sensitively care for their needs.

Give gifts to family and friends, not only on birthdays and holidays. Give for the sake of giving in ways that stretch you.

VISUALIZATION

Springtime is only a day—no, a breath—away from blossoming into summer. You are standing in the middle of a sparsely populated forest with patchwork sunlight scattering across the underbrush.

Begin to watch your breath. Become each breath. As you inhale, you find yourself growing in height. As you exhale, your feet become transmuted into roots, drawing in nourishment from the rain-drenched earth. Your hands are now many branches, housing both bird and squirrel. Imagine your body as a tree—sturdy and well-formed.

The earth, the sun and the rain have all treated you well. How can you thank them in return? Simply by being the most loving, caring tree you can be. Any deer seeking shelter from the wind will find it by nestling at the base of your trunk. Any bird needing rest will discover it in your leafy arms. Why, the very sun itself reserves a resting place in your highest branches when, at dusk, it wearies.

Inhale this attitude of selfless love and loving concern for others. And now, repeat the following affirmation.

AFFIRMATION

With friendship and compassion, I embrace my fellowman. In Spirit, I am one with all!

CHAPTER FIFTEEN

CORN:
"THE ENERGIZER"

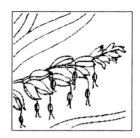

Zea mays
("cereal, or grass, maize")

"I just had to drop you a line to let you know how wonderful Corn is! I was pretty wigged out after the '89 San Francisco earthquake, feeling awfully drained, depressed, etc. And I had just started my new job the week before. Well, a few days after going on the Corn, I began to feel like a new person—and still do. I've been on a really strict diet, and have lost ten pounds. I have so much energy now, am feeling really positive and clear." —SG, Mountain View, CA

"I had been taking Corn for one week when I decided to move out of my old trailer to a new home. It was so helpful with the transition. Fast work!" —BA, Nevada City, CA

"I was going through a lot of changes—recently divorced, and having problems with my six-year-old son. 1 took Corn to enhance the growth already happening. I feel it is really working with me." —BC, Nevada City, CA

"The Corn seems to have worked better than is believable. I simply don't have to drag myself out of bed anymore—amazing for me." —ID, Flagstaff, AZ

"My wife is changing her job which would usually have her feeling uncertain and anxious about what will happen next. She gets miserable and stagnant with lots of contingent plans. She took two doses of Corn and says it had great effects. She has a lot more 'get up and go.'" —RC, Dallas, TX

"Corn allowed me to have the energy to release problems I had held inside. I was able to really talk to my boyfriend and clear the air between us." —CH, Munich, Germany

112

"Nothing is troublesome that we do willingly." —Thomas Jefferson

FLOWER/FRUIT/FOLKLORE

Corn is the only cereal crop with an American origin, and is widely found in tropical and subtropical regions throughout the world. Records indicate that a corn-like crop existed in Mexico over seven thousand years ago. In addition to being used as food by North American Indians, the Incas, Mayans, and Aztecs have employed it as a form of currency, jewelry, building material, and decorative art. An annual crop of the grass family requiring three to five months to mature, its female flowers with protruding "silk" are carried lower on the stems. The male flowers form short, feathery tassels at the top. Corn is considered one of the most balanced of starches. Though easy to digest, it is high in roughage, rich in magnesium and phosphorus, and strengthening to the brain and nervous system. Cornsilk, meal, kernels, and cob—all parts of the corn are medicinally beneficial in lowering cholesterol, regulating the bowels, strengthening the kidneys, and relieving skin rashes.

Quality: Mental Vitality
Message of Self-mastery: Energy; taking initiative in projects; enthusiasm; living fully in the moment; saying "Yes" to life's challenges; exuberant willingness; for new beginnings.
Pattern of Disharmony: Sluggishness; procrastination; unwillingness; blocked energy; unresponsiveness; dragging one's feet; resistance; lethargy; "Manana" state of mind; "passing the buck" attitude.

SPECTRUM PLACEMENT

Corn signifies the beginning of the Spectrum's masculine half. Birthed from Peach, it captures the masculine qualities of drive, expression, building, and the desire to achieve. This first house of Quadrant II expresses the energy of summertime and youthfulness with bountiful enthusiasm.

Summer, the warmest season of the year, possesses a certain fire, abundantly found in Corn's vitality.

POSITIVE APPLICATIONS

The positive Corn state exemplifies living fully in the moment. Instead of putting things off, we find we have the present in which to do them. Rather than living on auto pilot, we get ourselves in gear. The positive Corn state applies to getting jobs done, and more importantly, to an inner attitude of willingness and a commitment of energy to make needed psycho-emotional changes. One woman phoned to relate that, after taking one dosage of Corn in the evening, she didn't recognize her own reflection in the bathroom mirror the next morning!

"It's cloudy today. I think I'll stay home." "It's raining again—that really bums me out." What do both these statements have in common? Superficially, the weather. On a deeper level, both reflect a dependence on outer circumstances to make our lives work. If something so simple as weather contrary to our wishes can ruin our plans for the day, what would happen if true tragedy struck, such as a hurricane or an earthquake? Let's look at two reactions to what we might call "tragedies," one exemplifying the positive Corn state and the other, the negative Corn condition.

News coverage of the Los Angeles earthquake in January of 1994 poignantly documented its quake victims—the rich who had lost their mansions, their land, and everything but their lives. Close-up photos caught the anger, the disbelief, and the need to blame someone or something, all written into their faces. A pervasive "why me?" attitude prevailed, along with a need for the positive Corn state. In contrast to these quake victims, some friends of mine lost their home, which they had built themselves, in a forest fire years ago. At the time, their son was only weeks old. "Well," said my friend surveying the damage, "at least we won't have to deal with that leaky roof any more!"

What, then, is the difference between these two reactions to similar circumstances? Clearly, it's the nature of their energy. In one case, we see an attitude that life is "out to get us." In the other, the positive Corn state, we find the decision to put out the best possible energy to deal with circumstances as they are, reflecting a willingness to meet overwhelming odds with a spirit of inner joy.

The positive Corn state addresses both the quantity and the quality of energy. In other words, Corn may not inspire us to train for a marathon, but it will enhance the quality of the energy with which we face even small tasks. A good definition of Corn would be *life-affirming*. With this attitude, long put-off projects are welcomed, housework and routine chores become pleasant, and even Monday mornings are not so bad after all. The positive Corn state encourages us to do old things in new ways.

Corn is also strengthening when new projects are undertaken, such as starting a new job or considering one; a new school year, a move or going off to college, for both parent and child; or getting promoted at work.

NEGATIVE INDICATIONS

Negative Corn traits depict a lack of energy, expressed through lethargy, sluggishness, and—our worst enemy—unwillingness. This last quality is so detrimental to any flow of energy that we might well personify it as "the Unwillingness Monster." Surely we have all stood face to face with this beast at one time or another in our lives! Inarticulate and slovenly, he boasts a one-word vocabulary—"No." In an instant, he can sap our energy.

The word *vitality* stems from the Latin root, *vita*, meaning life. Life is synonymous with energy. The more vitality we own, the more enthusiasm we have for life.

Consider this scenario: It's Friday night, and you're beat from an especially trying work week. Nothing looks more inviting than a mindless night of television, garnished with a microwave dinner and a soft drink. That's all you have energy for anyway, and besides—you've earned it. Then the phone rings. It's a friend you haven't seen in years, inviting you to a concert headlining your favorite music group. Gosh, you hadn't even heard that they were in town! *Poof.* The lethargy's gone and you're ready in minutes for a night out.

Ruling out physiological causes, what better proof is there that low energy is a state of mind? And do couch potatoes really enjoy being that way? "After only one drop of Corn," wrote a mother of two young children, "I cleaned Katie's room and said, 'Let's make this a place of joy.' I was literally dancing while doing my housework. I do clean, but not with *this* good of an energy. It really changed me."

The negative Corn state also manifests as procrastination. "Why do today what you can put off till tomorrow?" as the saying goes. How easy it is to find a thousand reasons to rationalize our lack of energy! Consider the classic example of the smoker trying to quit. "Why, giving up smoking's the easiest thing in the world," Mark Twain once said. "I've done it hundreds of times."

THEME CHARACTERISTICS

"Energy and joy go hand in hand," is a saying that coins the essence of Corn. In this light, you will know Corn themes when you meet them because they are not subtle! Veritable storehouses of enthusiasm who sometimes seem to be running on fast-forward, their body language gives them away at a glance. Quick movements, animated gestures and facial expressions, and a voice that is just a notch too loud—these signs disclose the Corn theme. These people are mentally quick with responses and creative in their verbal comebacks. In their presence you will feel vivacious joy. You may be inspired to put out more energy in your own life—and good luck trying to keep up with them!

FAMOUS THEME PERSONALITIES

Henry Ford
Carol Burnett
Lucille Ball

Jay Leno
The Roadrunner
Frank Lloyd Wright
Herbert Hoover
The Wright Brothers
Charles A. Lindbergh

Henry Ford (1863-1947) is our Corn theme who presented to the public a moderately-priced automobile about fifty years ahead of its time. With new ideas and a new efficiency, his innovative application of the assembly line's mass production concept afforded many Michigan men what he called "a chance but no charity." There would be no handouts from this millionaire—just good honest wages for those who were willing to put out the energy.

Mr. Ford's great zest for life inspired a friend to describe him as one who "glided into a room like a panther with a twinkle in his eyes." A simple but energetic man who enjoyed dancing, friends, and taffy-pulling parties, Mr. Ford is responsible for the industrial miracle known as Ford Motors. "Start where you stand!" was one of his famous mottos, so perfectly capturing the Corn themes' indomitable vitality.

CONFESSIONS OF A CORN THEME: SONIA'S STORY

"Any personality quirks? Like that I'm addicted to coffee? Like that my fiancé says I do everything backwards?

"I am presently unemployed. Due to changes at my old job at a book distributors, there was the possibility that it wouldn't be that creative any more. So rather than having a job that was boring, I left. I just couldn't bring myself to the thought of going in every day and doing some monotonous thing over and over, day after day, while other people were doing really fun, creative things all around me. It's like, I just can't do this!

"So I decided to get a temporary job. I don't care what I do, I'll just find something fun. I'm not real super-picky, but I do need a job that's both heart-opening and mentally stimulating. I decided to move to a big city for awhile, to either get a job that pays a lot of money so that I wouldn't have to be there very long—or I could get a job that might not pay me a lot of money, but at least it would be something fun to do in the meantime until I find something better where my fiancé lives. I'm happy to be unemployed, I don't care!

"So I moved. Now I work for this company where I talk to clients all day long on the telephone. They call up and they say what they need for a caregiver, and I set up interviews. Yes, I like this job. It's mentally challenging, and it's a 'heart thing' because I'm dealing with people. People call up, they're in crisis, and I can help.

"Yes, I see myself as someone with energy. Vitality, no. I have a lot of energy, but I'm not particularly healthy, so I don't see myself as having vitality. Mental vitality, yes. Physical vitality, no. I have stamina, but it's not like I'm physically fit, so I don't feel like I have vitality.

"I like corn. I love corn! I've always liked corn; it's been one of my favorite vegetables. I love corn tortillas, corn chips, corn on the cob, cornbread—anything with corn in it. I've looked through that essence list, and corn always stood out."

WRAPPING IT UP

The Greek word *zea*, from the botanical name for corn, stems from the Greek *zao*, meaning "I live." Many North American Indian tribes considered corn a sacred plant, enacting the "corn dance ritual" to promote rain for their crops. Corn is a vegetable synonymous with life, even as Corn essence contains the quality of energy, without which life is impossible.

Do you remember the children's story, *The Little Engine That Could?* The train's affirmation, which he repeated again and again, was: "I *think* I can, I *think* I can!" So speaks Corn. This is the essence of will power, of decisions made, and of joyful follow-through with plans. But most of all, Corn's message is that, with mental vitality, we are "awake and ready" to tackle anything set before us.

CORN	Contrasted With:	Companioned With:
Apple	for energy that is specifically related to clarity	for a dynamic, unblocked flow of energy
Avocado	for a particular focus of energy	for focused energy
Coconut	for sustaining and completing tasks	for sustained and alert energy
Tomato	for facing weaknesses and fears	for an energy boost in the face of obstacles

POSITIVE EXPRESSIONS

Willing

Will-powered

Achievement-oriented

Energetic

Vitalized

Vigorous

Joyful

Zealous

Enthusiastic

Pioneering in spirit

Innovative

Initiating

Responsive

Creative

Life-affirming

NEGATIVE CONDITIONS

Wean-Exhausted

Lackluster

"Monday morning blahs"

Bored

"Couch potato"- prone

Stuck in a mental rut

Needing stimulants

Rationalizing

"Auto pilot" state

Low energy

Unwilling

Sluggish

Lethargic

Essence Enhancers

Go to new places for old routines—dining, shopping, entertainment.

Exercise regularly, join a health club, if necessary, for group support.

Build a brisk walk into your routine at the same time each day.

Take up a new hobby.

Try a new sport, either as a spectator, a player, or both.

Eliminate coffee, black tea, and excessive sugar consumption from your diet.

Visualization

The snows of a long winter are melting late into springtime in the higher mountainous elevations. Icicles metamorphose into well-fed streams, racing over aged rocks and occasional felled trees. This day paints itself in bold greens that shout and whisper of the initiation into a new season.

Summer bursts forth from the womb of a well-nourished spring, the earth now warmed by a hotter sun. The dance of new life, choreographed by a knowing Mother Nature, has begun. All living things grasp the present tense of action verbs. "Race," urges the river. "Fly!" cries the lark. "Flutter," whispers the butterfly. And the nouns, not wanting to be left by the wayside, shout from the very clouds. "Energy," says the breeze.

"Vitality," sings the mountain stream. "Freedom!" cries the wind.

All the elements of nature commune in harmony. And in this moment, eternity awakens.

Affirmation

With boundless energy I rise to greet the world!

CHAPTER SIXTEEN

TOMATO:
"THE PURPOSEFUL WARRIOR"

Lycopersicon esculentum
("tasty wolf-fruit")

"My seven-year old nephew really likes taking Tomato. It has definitely helped him get rid of nightmares." —*RB, Hayward, CA*

"I gained weight over the holidays. It really depressed me, so I took Tomato. It showed me that I am a fighter, and that I can face all my problems." —*UR, Plano, TX*

"I got very spacey and weak on a strict diet. Tomato really worked instantaneously. I felt 'back down to earth.'" —*KK, Nevada City, CA*

"Tomato acted like an anchor for me. It got me through a court experience about an inspection sticker for my car. I was able to deal with the facts, and not my anxiety. I was really steady."—*BS, Irving, TX*

"I was bogged down emotionally for so long. When I started Tomato, I awoke within myself to a state of clarity " —*HE, Menlo Park, CA*

"Everyone who comes to me for dental work says, 'I hate dentists, I hate to be here.' I use these drops for my patients, and they work great."

— *DS, Los Angeles, CA*

121

"Cowards die many times before their deaths; The valiant never taste of death but once."   —Shakespeare

FLOWER/FRUIT/FOLKLORE

This native of South America's lower Andes was introduced into Italy in the sixteenth century as the *pomodoro*, or "apple of gold." Once believed poisonous, it is still considered undesirable in the macrobiotic diet as a nightshade food. The tomato is a weak-stemmed herbaceous plant cultivated as an annual. The flower has a five-lobed, green calyx and five tiny yellow petals. Considered vegetables by cultivation, tomatoes are botanically classified as fruit. Like berries, they are pulpy and contain one or more seeds that are not stones. Tomatoes are rich in nutritional value, especially vitamin A, and are useful as blood and liver cleansers. Their potassium content is helpful for kidney ailments and hypertension. As a poultice, they relieve sunburn pain, while the powdered seeds make an excellent protein supplement.

Qualities: Mental Strength, Endurance
Message of Self-mastery: Knowing there is no failure, only another chance to succeed; courage; belief in oneself; invincibility; psychic protection; stability; remaining unaffected by the diverse energies of crowds and traveling; hope.
Pattern of Disharmony: Fear; weakness; nightmares; withdrawal; defensiveness; addictions; shyness; minor hesitation to severe terror; defeatist attitude; instability; for the stress of city life.

SPECTRUM PLACEMENT

Aptly named "the warrior essence," Tomato resides in Quadrant II's second house. Having gathered the accessed energy of Corn, it charges into battle against our fears, blocks, and weaknesses. In Tomato we see Corn's raw energy focused on the qualities of strength and endurance. Tomato blends the masculine half of the Spectrum with Quadrant II's get-up-and-go-for-it fire. Empowered and ready for battle, the warrior plans strategies, makes quick decisions, and then acts on them. Energy plus courageous action equals Tomato.

POSITIVE APPLICATIONS

Perhaps you have heard the Chinese quote: "Fear knocked at the door; faith opened it, and there was no one there." This is a Tomato maxim indeed! We might call Tomato "bottled ammunition." The positive Tomato condition can aptly be summarized in one word—empowerment. Where tests drag on for some duration, Tomato helps us to develop steadfastness. Tomato speaks of hope, victory, and the ensuing sense of celebration.

Tomato aligns us with the understanding that "quick is the succession of human events; the cares of today are seldom the cares of tomorrow, and when we lie down at night, we may safely say to most of our troubles, 'Ye have done your worst, and we shall meet no more." Thus wrote English poet Cowper, beautifully paraphrasing the essence of Tomato.

Tomato also vibrationally addresses future fears based upon past trauma, such as accidents, illness, or surgery—all of which are invasive experiences to the human body and aura. "I took Tomato first to help with my courage in dealing with a near-crippling motorcycle accident," recounted Todd. "It gave me added mental strength. I took it as the shock was wearing off and fear was trying to set in. But the fear never got a chance to develop."

For many people, travel can generate fear. Addressing states ranging from a sense of vulnerability and disorientation in foreign environments to the raw terror of air flights, Tomato Essence makes a welcome traveling companion. Even if we are only trekking to the nearest town for a day of errands, Tomato affords psychic protection and shields us from foreign or negative energies. "My new executive job required that I travel frequently," Virginia shared. "I am terrified of planes. In fact, you couldn't pay me to fly without a Valium and two plane-sized bottles of scotch! Tomato has replaced the sedative *and* the scotch. I take it the day of the flight, and then I'm fine."

NEGATIVE INDICATIONS

Tomato helps us battle anything from mildly annoying bad habits to major addictions. Webster defines addiction from the Latin root, *addicere*, as in "to give oneself up habitually to." Addictions may include substance abuse, smoking, overeating, wrong eating, harmful relationships, and even the seemingly insignificant difficulty in getting out of bed in the morning.

Through the repetition of wrong habits, we empower them. These wrong actions wear a groove in the brain, as it were, making them more difficult to overcome. "I know Tomato has helped me immensely," wrote a woman from Sacramento. "I ran out of it a few days ago, and can really tell the difference. It's enabled me to end a very abusive relationship with my boyfriend, despite his repeated attempts to reconcile with me. Could we safely assume that addictions are rooted in a basic, though misguided, desire for happiness? In some obscure way, the pursuit of addictive substances and actions is an attempt to achieve freedom from misery. Tomato empowers us with the positive vibrational experience of happiness from within, replacing a compulsive need that can eventually become physiological if continued.

Perhaps our battles are not always so grandiose. Maybe we're only trying to lose a few pounds. Still, the discouragement of failure—especially when repeated—creates a snowball effect that weakens our hope of succeeding in the future. When we hear ourselves saying, "Oh, I shouldn't," or "I'll start tomorrow"—somewhat similar to negative Corn's procrastination—we are verbalizing the negative Tomato state. What we are really saying is, "I secretly don't believe I have the strength to deal with this right now." Tomato helps us remember that "our strength grows out of our weakness," as the naturalist Emerson wrote over a century ago.

The negative Tomato state expresses itself as fears of both known and unknown causes: fear of weakness, of planes and cars, and the residual fear that follows accidents. It also addresses issues of repeated failure, of a lingering sense of inadequacy, and of faltering and uncertainty. Tomato also helps you to stand up for your own beliefs.

"I took Tomato for letting go of my firstborn when she went off to college," wrote Alena. "This was the first time that I was really clear that the essences do not negate your emotions, but rather help you to deal with them, and then let them go. This was my strength. I wasn't taking Tomato to prevent me from crying; I took it so that I would be centered in my tears, and then be able to let go of my daughter with joy."

When fear plays through the subconscious mind during sleep, we experience the negative Tomato state of nightmares. These "night demons" play over and over like a "broken record syndrome," unable to be released from the subconscious mind. Tomato replaces these night fears with a sense of inner knowing that they have "done their worst" and can then vanish as night into the day.

THEME CHARACTERISTICS

An unmistakable clue to the Tomato theme is a tone of voice that bespeaks purpose and conviction. In women's voices, you'll hear a slight gravelly tone. Tomato themes generally have excellent posture, with shoulders back to open the heart, and the chin parallel to the ground, as if poised to meet tests head on. Their bearing symbolically dares the enemy to "take his best shot."

One senses that these themes are not only poised for battle but open to its outcome as well, whatever it may be. Their mental qualities include readiness and a sense of the celebration of victory. Tomato themes are strengthening to be around. They inspire fearlessness in others, and support their ability to face monumental difficulties with courageous endurance.

Galileo
Jean-Luc Picard
Captain Kirk
James Bond
General Patton
The Ninja Turtles
Helen Keller
Rudolph Nureyev
Rachmaninoff
Andrew Jackson

Galilei Galileo (1564-1642), a Renaissance scientist and inventor, physicist and philosopher, epitomizes Tomato's essence. As one of many trials, financial difficulties forced the young Galileo to leave his university training in mathematics. Strengthened in true Tomato form by a lifetime of repeated setbacks, Galileo's discoveries through the simple telescope—a tool that he scientifically advanced—revolution-ized the medieval concept of the universe.

Galileo was labeled as a heretic by standards of the times. In 1633, he faced the Inquisition for his argument that the sun, not the earth, was the center of the universe. He barely escaped being burned at the stake for his doctrines. Galileo's life overflowed with Tomato-designed tests of superhuman strength and pioneering courage. Attacked for his world-transforming views, he held fast to his convictions, battling the opposition of an entire era. Ironically, this man of great vision spent the last years of his life in total blindness.

CONFESSIONS OF A TOMATO THEME: VICTOR SPEAKS

"I have a managerial position in a small company, so I'm kind of a lightning rod for a lot of issues. But there are also a lot of positive rewards to my work.

"I'm working on general strength and energy. It's good but needs to be stronger. This is a major area of focus for me, definitely. I feel the need for more balance. I think there's a lot of energy trying to come through. I need balance so that it can flow in the way it needs to.

"I've got a couple of relationship doozies out there to work on. One is that I'm feeling judged by someone. I need to de-personalize it. It makes me feel heavy, burdened, sad, and hurt. I deal with this test through endurance. When I feel speech is effective, I communicate. But there are a lot of times when I feel there's nothing to be done. I think the bottom line with all our tests is that we have to celebrate them—they are our liberation process.

"You know, it's funny. I went on a backpacking trip with four of my best friends. They took me out for my birthday. We went up into the Desolation Wilderness. We were sittin' around a fire in the middle of the night up in the high elevation and we started saying, 'Why are we here, in this life?' In other words, what did we come to learn? It seemed that each of us said exactly what the other people perceived as that person's best strength and quality. We were each individually putting it out as the very thing we came here to learn! So it's kind of interesting how that is.

"I always really miss the tomato fruits in the winter, and I'm sure that's in part a vibrational thing. I'm always eating salsa."

WRAPPING IT UP

There's an old Texan folk tale about a tomato plant: If it won't produce fruit, hit it with a broom, shake it up, and it will grow tomatoes. All humor aside, this pithy saying suggests that even the tomato plant is fearless! When we are afraid, our focus is on ourselves and we covet that fear. Our energy contracts. In the expansive Tomato state of courage, we can transmute this fear.

The message of Tomato lies in the realization that victory need not mean winning. Rather, it lies in our attitudes of strength and courage, which then magnetize success and the life-affirming quality of vigor.

TOMATO	Contrasted With:	Companioned With:
Almond	for self-control in overcoming immoderate habits and behaviors	for mental and emotional health and strength in battling excesses and addictions
Apple	for health-related fears	for confidence in the ability to overcome obstacles
Banana	for a quiet strength	for over-involvement and upset
Coconut	for perseverance through challenges and trials	for the long distance runner state of mind; particularly for tests of great length
Corn	for the energy to fight battles	for renewed energy when it lags
Lettuce	for agitated emotional states, including stagefright	for "calmness in the midst of batttle"

POSITIVE EXPRESSIONS

Strong

Courageous

Success-oriented

Steadfast

Empowered

Dauntless

Psychically protected

Hopeful

Invincible

Centered

Believing in oneself

Open

Readiness-oriented

Celebratory

Self-honest

Renewed while traveling

Stable

NEGATIVE CONDITIONS

Cowardly	Hesitating
Weak	Defeatist attitude
Nightmare-prone	Fearful of failure
Frail	Fearful of known causes
Anxious	Fearful of unknown causes
Quitter's attitude	Unstable
Shy	Lacking conviction

ESSENCE ENHANCERS

Read books—especially autobiographies—about heroes, heroines, and saints who have overcome monumental challenges in their lives through acts of strength and courage.

Make a list of your "failures" in one column. In the other, write the lessons you have learned and the qualities you have developed through those failures.

Write down your fears. Mentally play out the "worst-case scenario" with each one and say, "That wasn't so bad. I can handle it."

Any time you have a nightmare, try to remember it in detail and then offer it into a mental fire, much like the following visualization.

VISUALIZATION

Sit up straight, away from the back of your chair. Drop your shoulders back to expand your chest, your chin parallel to the ground. Place your hands comfortably at the juncture of the upper legs and torso. With eyelids closed, relax your eyes and let your gaze, like a lazy trail of smoke, drift upward. Allow your breathing to be deep and regular.

Imagine in your mind a crackling fire, blazing in its varied stages—first, the match catching the crumpled paper, followed by the burning of dry twigs and, as the fire spreads, the thin kindling. Then visualize the smaller logs igniting, pockets of sap making snapping sounds as a slight draft spreads the flames to larger wood stumps at the base of the fire.

Into this fire, mentally cast all fears. One by one, name them, tossing them into the flames. Feel that every cell in your body is purified of the poison of fear, and awakened as never before to the bright light of courage. Every crackle of the log is a new burst of that courage. Each shooting blaze is an affirmation of the fiery warrior within you, now and forever at your command.

AFFIRMATION

With strength and courage, I face all my trials!

CHAPTER SEVENTEEN

PINEAPPLE:
"THE CONFIDENT ONE"

Ananas comosus
("hairy, tufted pineapple")

"I took Pineapple for questioning my work and how to contribute to others. I was also uncertain about my relationship with my wife. I was floundering, vacillating. After taking Pineapple, I felt a real reassurance that I'm on the right path. I was convinced of the lightness of what I *am* doing. This knowledge gave me more power."

—*TM, Dallas, TX*

"Pineapple has greatly helped raise my feeling of personal power."

—*MS, Mesquite, TX*

"On of my clients is a vivacious, well-to-do, fun-loving woman. She said that she felt she wasn't good enough. After taking Pineapple, she returned and said that she knew herself, and had resolved her self-doubt."

— *IT, Vienna, Austria*

"Pineapple was chosen for me through kinesiology. I took the essence for one month. Within that month, I felt more confident and finally got the raise I felt I deserved. It amounted to ten thousand dollars! This was a surprise even to my boss, who said he hadn't asked for that much. I think the essence has helped me feel stronger. "

—*IK, San Jose, CA*

"Well, I was feeling nervous about getting up and giving a talk in front of several hundred people. Someone had left me a bottle of Pineapple, so I started taking it. I noticed that I felt better. And to my amazement, I did a great job with the class." —*PV, Nevada City, CA*

*"Every man has in himself a continent of undiscovered character.
Happy is he who acts the Columbus to his own soul."* —Sir J. Stevens

FLOWER/FRUIT/FOLKLORE

A South American native, this tropical fruit also grows in Hawaii, Malaysia, Australia, and South Africa. The pineapple is actually a collection of smaller fruits, with each of the cactus-like hexagonal sections marking a botanically individual fruit. When flowering, it appears as a cluster of blossoms on a single stalk; bulbous pink and green blossoms grow in the crown of leaves. High in vitamins A and C, pineapples require fifteen to twenty months to ripen. They are a wonderful digestive aid and also help with protein assimilation. Good for inflammation, especially after dental surgery and sports injuries, pineapple also thins the blood and helps to remove warts and corns.

Quality: Self-assurance

Message of Self-mastery: Content with self; career fulfillment; confidence; empowerment; strong sense of identity; wisdom; clarity with money issues; the ability to draw abundance.

Pattern of Disharmony: Inferiority complex; compares self to others; dissatisfaction with self; unhappy with job situation; undesired unemployment; an overbearing nature; a pushy personality; inability to choose a career and/or stick with it.

SPECTRUM PLACEMENT

Personal power and dynamic growth, like forest fires of character qualities, burn rampant through Quadrant II. Pineapple occupies this Quadrant's third house, or midpoint, where these qualities are most strong. Fed by the fearlessness of Tomato and about to be softened by Banana's humility, Pineapple stands out as the essence of those who know themselves—their talents, strengths, and their impact on others.

POSITIVE APPLICATIONS

An individual in the positive Pineapple state goes to himself for a second opinion. And why not? It will be as reliable as the first. Clarity, strength, and wisdom are the pinnacles of Pineapple. Here we see an extremely magnetic and charismatic expression of energy. Public speakers, politicians, actors, and people in the limelight are generally strong in positive Pineapple characteristics. The glamour of their achievements and the glare of their mistakes catch the public eye with equal impact.

Pineapple is the ideal essence for identity crisis during the teenage years ("I don't like myself"); for mid-life crisis ("Who am I *now?*"); or for any sudden or dramatic change in life that leaves us not quite knowing who we are. Pineapple vibrationally teaches us to know and to like ourselves, leading to our becoming supremely likable in the process—and to others as well.

Pineapple comes to the rescue when confidence fails us. "I was in a serious car accident a couple of years ago," Debbie recalled." From that time on, even as a passenger, my stomach would end up in my throat. I took Pineapple for two months, especially when the fear arose. The Pineapple allowed me to tell myself, 'You *know* what you have to do.' It allowed me to go through with it." Pineapple is the essence for self-assurance, meaning tested faith in our Higher Self.

NEGATIVE INDICATIONS

The negative Pineapple state makes itself known through flamboyancy and the flaunting of every quality *but* humility. Individuals trapped in this condition will verbally back you into a corner. They are loud and overbearing, the topic of conversation usually revolving around themselves or their ideas—political, environmental, or even metaphysical. You may not be able to get a word in edgewise, so be prepared to just listen! Instead of having a lot of character, the negative Pineapple person *is* a character.

Paradoxically, this type of behavior is often symptomatic of an inferiority complex. The negative Pineapple state may also manifest as its opposite, shyness. Here we see the wallflower at the party, standing at the back of the room staring down at his feet. "Self-assuredness is big issue for me," Paul admitted. "Almost immediately I felt results from Pineapple. I was less preoccupied with understanding myself and less worried about others' judgments."

Then there's the job arena. Doubting our abilities, dissatisfied with skills, and preoccupied with our shortcomings—these qualities contribute to an unhappy work environment. When asking for a raise, isn't the real question, "Am I worth it?" Pineapple is the essence for money issues. We see in the negative Pineapple state a self-fulfilling prophecy of defeat in which we might feel underpaid; unrecognized for our achievements, which may indeed be fine; unable to secure the raise we feel we deserve; or unappreciated by our superiors.

These circumstances are often mere reflections of our own poor self-image. How can we blame the law of magnetism for drawing to ourselves precisely that which we broadcast out to the world? We should, rather, applaud it for its consistency and thank it for such a prompt vibrational RSVP!

THEME CHARACTERISTICS

Pineapple themes transmit to others a strong sense of their own inherent "okay-ness." This theme in men makes them dashing; in woman, impressive. Pineapple themes inspire confidence and ennobling qualities through their example. In speech, they are direct and loud, though not unpleasantly so. "Having a way with words," they will charm, impress, and impact. These people are born leaders.

You will never call a Pineapple theme "what's-his-name." Distinctively eye-catching if not physically attractive, these themes possess a commanding presence and are easily spotted in a crowd. Wonderfully entertaining and engaging, they are the life of the party.

Their bigger-than-life quality, as though they are somehow amplified, is refreshing.

Over many years of consultations, I have observed an interesting distinction about the distinguished Pineapple. It applies as a theme essence more frequently than a plot remedy. True to its center-stage nature, it chooses not to be lost in the crowd of plot essences. Pineapple's is a solo, not a choral, voice.

FAMOUS THEME PERSONALITIES

John Fitzgerald Kennedy

Colonel William
Reiker

Lwoxana Troi

Bugs Bunny

Madonna

Mohammed Ali

Sean Connery

Demi Moore

Miss Piggy

Descartes

The son of a self-made businessman, JFK followed in his father's footsteps. About as Pineapple-ish as they come, this thirty-fifth United States president cut a dashing personal image in the eyes of the media, limelighted by a handsome family. A hero in Naval action during World War II; a Pulitzer Prize winner for his biography, *Profiles In Courage;* a renowned orator, admired by statesmen and common men alike: these are clues to his exemplary Pineapple theme nature. This outstanding president is acclaimed for many accomplishments as well as a few glaring foreign policy failures. For Pineapple's successes and failures alike are monumental, and may raise eyebrows, and tempers, at the same time.

Suffice it to say that both Kennedy's life and his passing were noteworthy. Assassinated at forty-six years of age in 1963, his death and four-day funeral were witnessed by millions of teary-eyed onlookers through unprecedented television coverage. Although his life was cut short, the deathless, Peach-like words of Kennedy's Inaugural Address have shaped the pillars of our nation: "And so, my fellow Americans, ask not what your country can do for you—ask what you can do for your country."

CONFESSIONS OF A PINEAPPLE THEME: JOYCE'S STORY

"Mentally, I'm intelligent, and I think people see that. I have a measure of self-confidence, but certainly not complete. If you line people up by the millions, I'll be on the self-confident end of human beings, but I have much insecurity. I think it might have a lot to do with my upbringing. Just the fact that every time I felt something from within, it wasn't corroborated without. And that can turn on you after you just hear it over and over. So you doubt yourself. But I definitely can tell you that if I feel guided in something, you can't budge me from it because I get it from inside. See, it's the things that are inside that I can trust. On the inside, I'm very self-assured if I feel something.

"My father was in the military. I loved it. I didn't mind moving—I loved the travel. I went forward to make new friends each time. I love the military—supporting the nation, feeling loyal, feeling proud to be an American, proud to uphold the ideals of what our country stands for in myself. The other side of the military is the fighting, harming, destruction, stiffness, rigidity. I've never been stopped at the point of just being willing to take discipline. I'm definitely not a follower.

"I have made lots of enemies in my life, and that hurts me greatly. I care deeply, and I do want to be in good relationship and harmony with people, but I'm not seen in that way. I feel misunderstood. Most people can only take a little bit of me!"

Wrapping It Up

The pineapple fruit requires about two years to mature. Likewise, its psychological quality of self-assurance often warrants many years of ripening. This fruit has a distinctive taste; we either like it or we don't. Even in a fruit salad it stands out, just as a Pineapple theme makes himself known in a crowd. The fruit, like the person, vibrationally conveys, "This is who I am."

"This above all," immortalized Shakespeare, "to thine own self be true." How timelessly this quote summarizes Pineapple. In knowing ourselves, we know truth; and in that knowledge, we become truly free.

PINEAPPLE	Contrasted With:	Companioned With:
Banana	for a quiet self-knowing	for balance between inner knowledge and outer expression
Strawberry	for a sense of self-worth; freedom from guilt and self-blame	for strength of character and a well-integrated, functional personality

Positive Expressions

Honest	Clear-minded
Content with self	Outspoken
Fulfilled by career	Strong character
Confident	Self-assured
Powerful	Strong sense of identity
Wise	Knowing limitations
Comfortable with money	Abundance-oriented

NEGATIVE CONDITIONS

Tending toward an inferiority
  complex
Comparing self to others
Feeling judged
Dissatisfied with self
Outrageous
Imposing
Pushy
Loud
Overbearing

Obnoxious
Career-indecisive
Unhappy with job
Unemployed
Shy
Proud
Tactless
Uncomfortable with money
  issues
Stuck in poverty-consciousness

ESSENCE ENHANCERS

Spend time with Pineapple themes, or with people you know who are successful.

Read about famous people, or watch movies about their lives—inventors, leaders, political figures, and athletes.

Go to performances by solo artists who have achieved a measure of greatness and recognition.

Develop on deeper levels those skills and talents in which you already excel.

Anytime you find that you are comparing yourself to others—stop!

VISUALIZATION

It is a warm summer day. Were it not so early, the heat would have set in and made the hike before you even more strenuous. You survey the mountain from its base, and mentally brace yourself for a rugged morning climb. Your daypack holds some high carbohydrate snacks and a canteen of water filled from a spring at camp. A few deep breaths, and you're off. The trail proves well worn and solid under your hiking boots. Two pairs of socks should prevent any blistering. You are confident; all is ready.

The ascent is steady, the scenery varied and interesting. First you traverse a cool forest of hardwoods, the dew barely covering patches of moss. Then the trees thin out and the landscape grows sparse. The trail is much dryer now, and covered with pieces of brown and gray shale. The sun beats down in a familiar and friendly way. The ascent steepens. No matter, you know you can do it. Free from all doubt, confidence matches your every step.

You are breathing harder now, feeling your leg muscles challenged more deeply as you climb over rocks and large boulders. Although the hike has grown more difficult, you meet it without resistance. Endorphins flow within you like a cool stream, washing into your inner sight a great sense of power and self-knowing.

You pause on the trail and breathe in the quality of self-assuredness—owning it, honoring it, realizing it. One with the mountain, the sun, the trail, you inhale the sweet breeze of a triumphant climb.

Affirmation

I move with confidence through the graceful dance of life!

CHAPTER EIGHTEEN

BANANA:

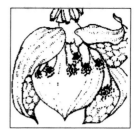

Musa paradisiaca
("banana fruit of paradise")

"THE HUMBLE SERVANT"

"Yesterday, after taking Banana, I reacted calmly to my husband's demands. 'Don't you think you should pot that plant now?' he asked twice. Instead of reacting and getting angry, I stayed calm, answered him, and continued reading my book." —*JP, Dallas, TX*

"Banana helped me deal with both personal and impersonal issues— financial and political, respectively. I have more energy to 'go with what happens.' I feel more whole. Also, I was having problems with my husband. Now I let him react without my reacting back."
—*UK, Plano, TX*

"My friend teaches elementary school. I felt that she needed a lot of help. She has twenty-three kids—sixteen are boys. She sprays her class room with Banana. It definitely helps." —*GK, Newbury, OR*

"My strong-willed five-year-old daughter insisted on staying home from our long-planned vacation to Gram's so that she could attend her best friend's birthday party. She was proud and resolute in her decision to stay, despite the inconvenience it would cause to the other family members. Immediately after I gave her a drop of Banana, she looked up at me and said, 'I think we should go to Gram's because we haven't seen her in a long time.'" —*KK, Sacramento, CA*

"I was craving bananas. When I took Banana Essence, the craving quit. I took it when I had trouble calming down to meditate. It always helps, it stills my mind." —*RD, Hayward, CA*

"Humility, that low sweet root, from which all heavenly
virtues shoot." — Thomas Moore

FLOWER/FRUIT/FOLKLORE

The name, *Musa paradisiaca,* includes the edible varieties and alludes to the ancient myth that bananas existed in the garden of Eden. *Musa sapientium* translates as "fruit of the wise men." Wild bananas date back to prehistoric times and are now cultivated in all parts of the tropics as well as in the region from India to New Guinea. This seedless fruit grows on a giant herb and not a tree, with a stem of overlapping leaves. The plant reaches a height of ten to thirty feet. A flowering stem emerges at the plant's apex carrying the male flowers. Higher on the stem are the female flowers, or hands, which hide twelve to sixteen bananas each. Bananas are rich in fiber. Their high potassium content aids the muscular system and they are helpful in feeding the natural acidophilus bacteria of the intestines. The peels also help with migraines, hypertension, skin sores, and rashes.

Quality: Humility Rooted in Calmness ⟵
Message of Self-mastery: Calmness; self-honesty; self-forgetfulness; ability to step back and observe, non-reactiveness; not getting caught up in negativity; understanding that "what goes around comes around"; for healthy distance from people and circumstances; objectivity.
Pattern of Disharmony: Focusing on oneself; anxiety; negative attachment; loss of perspective; "can't see the forest for the trees"; clouded judgment; nervousness, a quarrelsome nature; false pride; for a deep-seated need for recognition; for "going bananas."

SPECTRUM PLACEMENT

Banana, inhabiting Quadrant II's fourth house, is the natural successor to Pineapple. Whereas Pineapple is the magnetic speaker, Banana is the dynamic listener. While Pineapple occupies center stage, Banana is "the strong, silent type," or the "man of few words" and for this very reason oft misunderstood or overlooked.

Quadrant II's fire burns steadily in Banana, as do the masculine qualities of reason and detachment. You may be wondering what Banana, so soft and gentle, is doing in this Quadrant and in the masculine half of the Spectrum. Make no mistake: humility is a quality of enormous strength. If you want to put Banana to the test, try withdrawing from an argument when you think you are right!

POSITIVE APPLICATIONS

As St. Francis de Sales noted: "Nothing is so strong as gentleness, nothing so gentle as real strength." These words capture the essence of Banana. True strength has no need to boast of itself. Genuine fortitude is gentle, and quiet. Its proprietor knows that it knows and that is enough. Humility's strength, then, is its action as a vehicle for a higher power to manifest through us instead of being the end result in and of itself. A great saint was once praised for being humble. "How can there be humility, " he asked, "when there is no sense of ego?"

Banana's greatness lies in its ability to help us step back, or out of the way altogether, in circumstances that would otherwise snag us—a quarrel with the spouse, a confrontation at work, or feeling out of sorts and on the verge of anger or frustration. When we are able to remain nonreactive in the face of confrontation, we are in the positive Banana state. When we take a farsighted view of our problems, we are again expressing the gentle strength of this essence. One man recounts, "After the first night on Banana, I felt like my past was wiped clean and forgiven. I have an easy and soft feeling inside now."

Melanie relates: "I have been dealing with a difficult mental/emotional state for three years. It involves a broken heart—a loss of love, resulting in depression, insecurity, melancholy, and self-pity. I experienced Banana's qualities of humility and calmness as aids to greater detachment and started seeing my problem as less important, thinking of others first.

"At first on Banana, it felt like I'd taken a Valium. I had a distinct feeling of just rolling with the punches. After one week it seemed to have done its job because it no longer felt important or on my mind to take it. Even my coworker remarked on the change—there was nothing *but* Banana that I could attribute it to. I felt very detached all week. I have learned some valuable new habits from Banana."

NEGATIVE INDICATIONS

The negative Banana condition is one that we have all experienced at one time or another. Honest pride in our accomplishments is harmless and is, in fact, healthy. But false pride is another. To lose sight that true achievements come to us from a higher level of inspiration—the superconscious, mentioned in the Coconut chapter—creates a block in our energy flow, much like damming up a stream.

The negative Banana state is exhibited as the need to be right; the I-told-you-so attitude; the desire to add our two cents when what we're really after is having the last word. These attitudes—anxiety, nervousness, and a quarrelsome nature—are the foes of true calmness. Through Banana's quiet strength we are able to say, "Yes, maybe I was wrong"—or to say nothing at all where words would only prove inflammatory.

We have all experienced someone trying to "get our goat," the goat symbolizing our peace of mind. To give in to negative emotions by getting angry or upset, even righteously so, means we have lost. Instead, we have only succeeded in filling our bodies with biochemical poisons manufactured by negative emotions. If repeated often enough, this harmful pattern inscribes into our cells the blueprint for disease and the need for Banana.

THEME CHARACTERISTICS

The Italians have an expression for proud people—"sotto il naso"— referring to those who view the world "beneath the nose." We, too, describe the prideful as those who look down their noses at others.

Thus the humble, prayerful posture of the Banana theme belies his true nature—his head slightly lowered, though not downcast, and an almost imperceptible bow to the spine.

These are soft-spoken people—you may need to ask them to speak up—as well as especially good listeners. Through their own inner stillness, they draw to themselves quiet environments. Being in their presence helps others to see the larger realities around them. Veiled in inconspicuousness, Banana themes are Pineapples' polar opposite. Banana themes are easily overshadowed by the Pineapple and Corn themes of this world. The very quality in which they are so great is their littleness.

FAMOUS THEME PERSONALITIES

Gandhi •
Luther Burbank
George Washington Carver
Derek Bell
Frank Laubach
Linus from "Peanuts" cartoons
Sarada Devi
Gerhart Tersteegen

History records Mohandas Karamchand Gandhi (1869-1948), called Mahatma or "great soul," as the father of independent India. This humble statesman, a perfect Banana theme, demonstrated that the best leader is he who serves. Gandhi practiced and exemplified a philosophy of nonviolence called *satyagraha*, meaning truth, or soul force. Identifying himself with the Indian caste of the untouchables, he wore only a loin cloth and traveled in third-class trains. What better testimony to his resolute humility? (Yogananda, by the way, met with Gandhi in 1935; he described the statesman as a hundred-pound saint who "radiated physical, mental and spiritual health.")

Gandhi embodied a humility that superseded the ego-quality of self-protectiveness. In fact, true to his Banana theme of disidentification with his own body and mind, he once refused anesthetics for an appendectomy, chatting with friends during the operation! In his own words: "All that I can in true humility present to you is that Truth is not to be found by anybody who has not got an abundant sense of humility. If you would swim on the bosom of the ocean of Truth you must reduce yourself to a zero." Of Gandhi's many Banana-like qualities, perhaps the most striking was his simple gesture after being mortally wounded—a hand gently raised in blessing and forgiveness of his assassin.

CONFESSIONS OF A BANANA THEME: ROY SPEAKS

"Well, I guess I wouldn't know what to talk about. What would you like me to say? I told you I'm not a super talker. I have a lot of quirks, though, but none of them are particularly interesting. I get upset with myself over my failings. I hit my head against the wall—things like that. That's probably the worst of my faults. And this is probably not going to make a good story!

"I don't remember my childhood. I thought it was reasonably happy, that's what everybody told me. I remember having a pleasant time, don't remember any bad things. I had a wonderful loving family, and I had more than I should have of everything.

"I did construction work until about three years ago. I work at the computer now and talk to people a lot. Operations Manager is my title in a business that produces equipment for renewable energy systems.

"It's probably tricky for anybody to talk about his emotions. I do tend to overreact a lot. I guess I'm emotional. I deal with this by leaving the scene of the action for awhile. This gives you a chance to think in a better perspective. Then I feel better and get the chance to see things clearly. I don't overreact to people too much generally, but more to situations. Some people are real cool and calm—my boss, for example. You could drop a bomb near him and he'd be fine. If something like that happens to me, I get excited and usually say something that I wish I could have taken back. But by then it's too late—the moment to act correctly is gone. This is a major issue for me, but I'm doing better at it.

"The one quality I would most like to perfect is more calmness, which means being less emotional. You need emotions, but emotional extremes are what I mean. I manage to pull it off most of the time. For myself, I try to listen to others. In fact, I've had people tell me that I listen to them really well. Sometimes I think I listen too much. If I'm going to err, I'd rather err on that side even though it takes up too much of my time.

"Am I humble? Let's put it this way—I have a lot of reasons to be humble because I'm not particularly good at anything. I mean, you'd have to be red-hot at something to be humble about it. If you didn't excel, you'd have nothing to be humble about."

Wrapping It Up

The female banana flower is a deep shade of purple, its petals thick and firm. Growing like little children under the protection of its hands are a dozen or so pale bananas. The more they ripen and absorb weight, the lower the flower bows on its stalk, closely resembling one bowed in prayer yet dressed in the purple robes of a king. Symbolized in the flowering banana plant we see both the nobility of being humble and the humility of true greatness.

Banana allows us a detached view of life—and of ourselves. "The sufficiency of my merit is to know that my merit is not sufficient," admitted St. Augustine. In the positive Banana state, there is no questioning of our worth or excellence, no belittling of our capabilities. What, we would argue, exists to question or belittle? There is, however, in addition to our worthiness, credit given to the Creator as the source of all calmness and the origin of true greatness.

BANANA	Contrasted With:	Companioned With:
Almond	for calmness through control of desires	for the wisdom to discriminate beyond the level of emotions and desires
Lettuce	for calmness of emotions	to be an observer of one's life and not get caught up in disturbing emotions
Strawberry	for a healthy self-image	for seeing dysfunction as a part of the process toward integration as lessons are learned
Tomato	for breaking negative habit patterns	for tests designed to pull you off center, drawing you into emotional involvement

POSITIVE EXPRESSIONS

Humble

Gentle

Modest

Calm

Strong

A good listener

Verbally abstemious

Detached

Clear-thinking

Non-reactive

Peace-loving

Dignified

Greatness of character

Surrendering

Quiet

NEGATIVE CONDITIONS

Shy
Obstinate
Lacking in clarity
Nervous
Quarrelsome
Drawing conflict
Overly attached
"Going bananas"
Needing to be right

Reactive
Uptight
Clouded in judgment
Falsely proud
Defensive
Easily upset
Arrogant
Opinionated

ESSENCE ENHANCERS

Read about the lives of famous Banana theme personalities.
Meditate.

If you find yourself involved in an argument, say to your opponent, "Maybe you are right." Release the need to be right, and be open to what you can learn from the experience.

Study one of the martial arts, and learn to work with nonviolent flows of energy flows.   *Joseph*

VISUALIZATION

A gentle surf on the tropical shore rhythmically drums its fingers on the shell-strewn beach. As an exercise in consciousness, identify yourself with the sand. "Tap, tap, tap," reiterate the waves. Now allow your consciousness to recede from the beach that is presently upstaged by a five-star sunset of ever-changing hues. Observe the deep reds and kingly violets weave soft patterns in the quiet sky.

"Who am I?" you ask the wave-stirring wind. "Who is asking?" the wind, in question form, replies. You set the question aside like a toy sand pail and dive into the waves. Imagine yourself floating, raft-like, upon them. Play with the thought of becoming a wave. The rivulets to your left and right for miles are like brothers and sisters. You frolic together on the ocean of life. Become the littlest wave possible. And now become merely the salty froth on that wave.

Foam on one small wave in a great big ocean? How little you are! How tiny, and humble. And how little "you" matter anyway. A wave of great calmness washes over you in the realization of your little part in the oceanic drama of creation.

AFFIRMATION

I am a ripple of calmness among towering waves of egotism on life's restless sea!

CHAPTER NINETEEN

FIG:

Ficus carica
("common orchard fig")

"THE NON-DISCIPLINARIAN"

"I've seen Fig help my clients who have Candida and strict diets. It loosens up the energy around their ailments and helps them work with their restrictions without such grim determination."

—*NB, Nevada City, CA*

"I put a few drops of Fig in my client's massage oil for tight shoulders. At first she thought she didn't need it till reading about the emotional qualities of Fig. She commented later that she felt herself more relaxed in her dealings with people, and that she was really helped by just those few drops in one application."

—*CS, Menlo Park, CA*

"I had been very tense when I took Fig. It made me very tired because I finally relaxed."   —*SR, Vienna, Austria*

"I took Fig for difficulty in making a decision. Shortly after, the issue seemed to dissolve. Clarity replaced it, along with a feeling of internal rightness."   —*SL, Camptonville, CA*

"I never talk about how I really feel. After taking Fig, I was able to tell my boyfriend how sad I was that he didn't want to marry me. He was surprised and open. He really listened to me."

—*NU, Eltangen, Germany*

"Do what you can with what you have, where you are."
—Theodore Roosevelt

FLOWER/FRUIT/FOLKLORE

Figs, native to western Asia, are grown in Asia Minor, Greece, Italy, Algeria, Portugal, and California. A member of the mulberry family, the fig is a deciduous shrub or small tree of thirty feet. The tree produces three to five palmately lobed leaves per stem and tiny stem-like buds. It is these buds that are used to prepare flower essences, since the actual flowers grow inside the fruit. Many tiny seeds and a soft pinkish-white pulp are enclosed within the fruit's thin skin. Due to their high sugar content, figs are great energy-producers. They are rich in calcium and laxative value from their mucin and pectin content. Bland in taste, the fresh fig is an emollient that can be used externally to soothe or protect the skin. Figs also help relieve sore throats, boils, and chronic joint inflammation.

Qualities: Flexibility and Self-acceptance
Message of Self-mastery: Sense of humor; fluidity; ability to "go with the flow"; at ease with self and others; self-liberating; energy to move forward in life; relaxation; for setting healthy boundaries; ability to "roll with the punches."
Pattern of Disharmony: Rigidity; tension; an uncompromising nature; difficulty with change; unrealistic expectations of oneself; fanaticism; self-limiting; too strict a sense of discipline; for over-extending oneself; self-dominating; suppression of faults; trying too hard; self-martyrdom; judgmental of self.

SPECTRUM PLACEMENT

Fig occupies Quadrant II's fifth and last house. Like Banana, it possesses a mixture of gentleness and strength—the strength born of flexibility and the ability to go easy on ourselves.

Consider the skin of a ripe fig—deep-hued purple, fleshy, and easily bruised, as if it were both youthful and aged at the same time. Metaphorically, Fig is Quadrant II's perfect closure. Enriched with the energy of youth, it serves as a transitional essence to Quadrant III's characteristics of autumn and middle age.

POSITIVE APPLICATIONS

The positive Fig state is expressed as flexible, fluid, and adaptable energy. Easy to get along with and open to new ideas, individuals in the positive Fig state make great companions. Arbitrators, umpires, emperors, and judges—all are fitting Fig-like roles. Ask them for help in making decisions. Able to see both sides of the picture, they can dive into their bag of wisdom without inhibitive rules blocking their natural understanding. These are classic "go with the flow" people.

Fig supports the development of discrimination without judgment, and clear observation without criticism. Feeling comfortable about yourself—your appearance, your daily habits, and your outlook on life—is the voice of Fig. The ability to accept both your strengths and weaknesses, and your victories and mistakes, is the echo of Fig. Living in the positive Fig state allows us to adapt to changes, ranging from sudden to long anticipated. And since change and growth are inherent to the human condition, we all need Fig's remarkable support at one time or another. This essence exemplifies a state of relaxation—the perfect balance between discipline and flexibility.

NEGATIVE INDICATIONS

The negative Fig state manifests as too many self-created rules that confine instead of freeing us. Negative Fig forces us to live in a little box of "should's" and "have-to's." It is said that too many rules kill the spirit. Perhaps we have created ideals that we cannot live up to. Maybe we have placed unrealistic expectations on ourselves that have only constructed walls of tension and frustration.

It is important to note the difference between Fig and Date. Whereas we project Fig's perfectionist attitude onto ourselves, the judgmental attitude of the negative Date condition is aimed at others. The negative Fig is self-critical; negative Date is critical of others.

Fanaticism, dogmatism, and many other "isms" are symptomatic of the negative Fig state. Fanaticism can easily find fertile soil in the garden of daily habits, diets, and religious beliefs. Its fruits, though, are always the same—mental rigidity. "I have so many food allergies that there's very little I can eat without having reactions," Cheryl lamented. "I have to deal with bloating, constipation, and skin rashes. When I took Fig, I noticed that my symptoms were greatly lessened. With this encouraging sign, I've been eating a greater variety of foods."

Indeed, diet is a well frequented arena for the indication of Fig. We live in a society where obesity is a serious health problem, not to mention the opposite extreme of eating disorders such as bulimia and anorexia. Obsessed as we are with the stick-like figures adorning glamour magazines, it's no wonder we're confused! As the New Age saying goes, "denial" ain't just a river in Egypt. Fig, then, not only works with excessive food intake; it also helps those on restrictive health diets to relax with their prescribed programs.

THEME CHARACTERISTICS

Fig's ability to take things in stride gives these themes a precise way of walking. "I choose to walk this way," they seem to be saying, holding their bodies in strict obedience to an orderly mind.

Fig themes make wonderful orators who can inspire us with both high, and attainable, ideals. They are articulate in speech, at times correcting themselves or searching for just the right words. You'll hear them say, "What I mean is. . . " or, "What I'm trying to say is. . . " Listen closely to their laughter; it will be interesting as well as distinctive.

These people are comfortable with themselves and wear their bodies like favorite, well-worn but stylish outfits. Their magnetism vibrationally encourages others to be more self-accepting and less self-critical.

Famous Theme Personalities

Carolus Linnaeus
Iyengar
Adelle Davis
Henry Higgins
Meryl Streep
Dustin Hoffman
Queen Elizabeth I
George Bernard Shaw
Abraham Lincoln
Melvil Dewey

The man who first coined the term, *homo sapiens*, meaning "wise men," is Carolus Linnaeus. Only a serious Fig theme would go to the trouble of classifying every existing plant, animal, and microorganism! Linnaeus meticulously (a fitting Fig adjective) grouped all flowering plants by their number of stamens and pistils into a system called "binomial nomenclature." In so categorizing flowers and all living things, he made our world a little more orderly.

It is written that Linnaeus was a cheerful fellow with a Fig theme's sense of humor. He used to guide his students on nature walks through the Swedish countryside, announcing their discoveries of uncommon specimens with a blast of his trumpet. And although no records document his early life, we are probably safe in assuming that, as a child, he always put his socks away! In 1761, Linnaeus was knighted by the Swedish government. He then took the un-Latinized name of Carl von Linnee.

Confessions of a Fig Theme: Blair's Story

"Discipline is part of my nature. Since I was a child, it was always like that. In my youth, I took it to an extreme and I separated myself from others to keep my routine. When I did connect with people, I felt that I had to give up my discipline. This was not right for me. It caused a lot of pain because I wanted to be connected. Now I need to learn how to soften this aspect of myself and make my connection with the world. Even to realize this is not an easy thing to face. But at the same time, this will move me forward to break through my own limitations.

"I have a real schedule for my life and my meditation practices. I don't break my routine or my order to go to town or go to a movie. I am working on being more open to having more of a flow in my life—and this doesn't mean that I'm going to lose my discipline. I am learning that it is possible to be with other people, and to include them in my own reality and my own discipline without losing my sense of self. My fear is loss of self, loss of discipline. Having my own way is rigidity.

"Do I like figs? I love figs!"

WRAPPING IT UP

The fig tree, as mentioned earlier, bears no outer flowers. Its blossoms ripen within the fleshy-seeded fruit itself. This flower-within-the-fruit metaphor symbolizes the blossoming of our own internal rules with malleable, self-made guidelines rather than self-limiting iron bars.

Here's a perfect Fig story: One day, an army lieutenant decided to grill his troop with a pop quiz. "Soldier," he asked, "why is the butt of a rifle made out of walnut?" "Because, Sir, it's a hard wood." "Wrong," retorted the lieutenant. He then asked the next soldier, "Why is the butt of a rifle made out of walnut?" "Sir, because it is smoother than other wood." "Wrong," replied the lieutenant, his patience waning. Asking the third soldier the same question, the answer came: "Because it polishes better." The lieutenant shook his head and said, "You boys just don't get it. The correct answer is—because regulations say so."

When rules override practicality and common sense, we may be assured that we are trapped in the negative Fig state that is uncomfortably joyless at best. The positive message of Fig is found in a sense of humor; in being delighted and delightful; and in replacing the perfectionist's rigid idealism with the ingenuity to simply "make do." Or, to quote Roosevelt, to "do what you can with what you have, where you are."

FIG	Contrasted With:	Companioned With:
Almond	for wisdom through self-control and moderation	for flexibility, not laxity; for malleability while holding firm to healthful ideals
Avocado	for mindfulness	for seeing the bigger picture as well as details
Date	for being too hard on others	for balance through accepting oneself and others; acknowledging imperfections tolerantly
Strawberry	for guilt, sense of unworthiness	for self-acceptance and self-study without harmful judgment

POSITIVE EXPRESSIONS

Pliant

Adjustable to change

Adaptable

Disciplined in moderation

Flexible

Open-minded

Fluid

Articulate

Wise

Relaxed

Self-accepting

Having a sense of humor

Tolerant

Intuitive

Self-liberating

Able to set healthy boundaries

Self-guiding

NEGATIVE CONDITIONS

Unadaptable

Mentally rigid

Perfectionistic

Holding unrealistic ideals

Self-denying

Obsessive

Compulsive

Harsh disciplinarian

Overly serious

Tense

Fanatical

Dogmatic

Self-limiting

Self-critical

Condemning

Judgmental

Critical

Overly-disciplined

Inhibited

Inhibitive

ESSENCE ENHANCERS

Mentally note areas of your life where you are self-critical. Focusing on one area each week, consciously redefine yourself in positive and supportive ways.

Do yoga postures through the aid of a class, a book, or a good video.

Allow enough time in your daily schedule for relaxation and entertainment—anything from a leisurely walk to having friends over for dinner.

Read light fiction or humorous pieces every day.

VISUALIZATION

Summertime closes its doors in the face of autumn. The warm sunny days, like candy wrappers, are pinched at both ends by a new chill in the air. Sweaters at dawn and dusk are now a must. The leaves have not yet put on their new colors, but you can tell they're thinking about it. "What to wear?" you almost hear them muse. "A rusty red, perhaps? A grocery bag brown? This green has got to go!" Their sense of humor, stemming from complete acceptance of the changing seasons, makes you chuckle.

But dress they must for this most special event of their lives—the windborne descent from limb to ground. No matter that the trees' withdrawn life force relegates them to the category of vestige. Their final role is the fluttering, earthbound dance. At curtain call they will either be raked up into large piles on lawns where children will gleefully pounce on them, or quietly compost themselves to nourish their beloved mother trees in the timeless cycle of death and rebirth.

Ah, here comes the wind now, right on schedule! Mother Nature's arm sports no wristwatch; she knows by sixth sense when everything needs to happen. But very few people know the truth about the wind— that it is Mother Earth's breath. She blows and blows, like a child extinguishing festively lit birthday candles—over the mountains, through the mesas, and around the trees. Her wind-breath bends and bows; its strength lies in its flexibility. The wind plays by the rules—but it also knows when to break them.

You, too, are like the wind—strong yet gentle and disciplined yet malleable.

AFFIRMATION

I am relaxed and peaceful: I am one with all that is!

CHAPTER TWENTY

ALMOND:

"THE SELF-CONTAINER"

Prunus amygdalus
("almond-like plum tree")

"I took Almond for feeling too busy. I felt good and peaceful on it—also more open and relaxed."
—JL, Sandpoint, ID

"I used Almond while driving to town. It helped me stay calm and centered, and also to avoid being emotionally affected by the driving habits of others."
—RB, Walnut Creek, CA

"I was making the transition from ending a relationship to being single. I took Almond for feeling over-sexed, morning and night. It was too much. After one month on the Almond, my energy had changed. I experienced my sexuality differently—as though Almond helped bring together my spirituality and sexuality. What I mean is, I found the spirituality in my sexuality. No, sex is not over, I told myself—but Almond took it to a deeper level."
—GH, Vienna, Austria

"My oldest son, twenty-two years old, has a girlfriend. She is a student with much work to do and little time for socializing and romance. Since he was desiring sex more often than she, I offered him Almond. He was then able to match his drives to hers."
—IR, Vienna, Austria

"My client was working on abuse issues from a close relative in her childhood. Although married, she was also obsessed with thoughts of another man. She was both confused and unclear about leaving her husband, and reported that Almond was a real key to help her work through this very difficult situation."
—SC, Nevada City, CA

> *"Joy, temperance, and repose, slam the door on the doctor's nose."*   —Longfellow

FLOWER /FRUIT /FOLKLORE

The almond tree is also called *Prunus dulcis,* meaning sweet, pleasing, or delightful. Almond is the oldest known nut tree and a member of the rose family. Naturalized in Western Asia and Southern Europe, the small almond tree (which looks much like the peach tree) originated in the Near East, and now grows in a hundred varieties in South Africa, South Australia, and California. Its pink flowers—similar to, but larger than, peach blossoms—reach up to two inches in diameter, and grow in fascicles of one to three. The nuts ripen from a peach-like fruit. The almond nut is a seed without a shell, high in fiber, B vitamins, and eight of the nine essential amino acids—and calories too. Its protein content is legendary, and it is rich in bone-strengthening minerals and cholesterol-lowering mono-unsaturated fats. Almond oil aids skin problems; the milk soothes the lungs and throat.

Qualities: Self-control and Moral Vigor

Message of Self-mastery: Calmness of the mind; synchronicity of body/mind/spirit; sense of well-being and order; to avoid "burning the candle at both ends"; balance; moderation; wholesome sexuality; for being a sensitive partner in an intimate relationship.

Pattern of Disharmony: Over-indulgence in food or other substances/ activities; immoderation, causing minor to serious damage to body, mind, or nerves; sexual excess in thought or action; making wrong choices from the power of past habits; discontentment; uneasiness; for anger connected with sexual issues; frustration.

SPECTRUM PLACEMENT

Almond is our usher into Quadrant III. We continue in the masculine half of the Spectrum, signifying that these five essences possess strength, power, and the drive to build and accomplish. The third Quadrant symbolizes the personality ripening in wisdom much like a garden awaiting autumn's harvest. In its first house placement, Almond encapsulates the matured strength to say "no" to excess. Having learned Fig's lesson of balance, Almond portrays a healthy sense of self-control.

POSITIVE APPLICATIONS

Almond is the essence for self-control in all parts of our lives. This quality, unfortunately, is not a high priority in our culture where consumerism and materialism are so seriously valued. And yet what a priceless tool for well-being is discipline! Self-control means, simply, that we consider a choice of action rather than being bound to a reactive mode by the subconscious mind.

Almond, then, gives us greater awareness in our choices. In the relationship arena of sexuality, our self-control is a gift we can give to our partner. Sex has two distinct purposes—procreation, and communicating love. With Almond's attitude of "how can I serve you" instead of "what's in this for me," the sexual act becomes purified from self-seeking and self-gratification, and thus infinitely more beautiful and fulfilling. We are not body-bound slaves to our senses, says Almond—we are Spirit.

Almond also encapsulates the quality of moral vigor and stimulates that same quality within us. Do you want the power to rebound vigorously from every setback in life? To live more in your center? Don't think of the crunchy quality of the nut, but of the soothing, spiritual influence of the oil pressed from almonds.

And what of stress from the sense that there are not enough hours in the day—don't we all have twenty-four? In the positive Almond state, we are able to view our time differently—to be more in the present moment, calmly completing each task. "I took Almond for tension that created pressure and tightness in my diaphragm," Ursula said. "In thirty minutes, it was gone."

Robert, too, shared a helpful Almond story: "I recently had to go to the dentist to have an area worked where a filling had fallen out. I took Almond and did the affirmation. I noticed I was able to relax deeply while in the chair. Though the area being drilled was sensitive from an exposed nerve, I found that I was able to remain calm and detached from the sensation."

Almond is also an excellent remedy for dancers. Yogic tradition speaks of being "centered in the spine," that place in the astral body from which our energy radiates. Dance, when most beautiful and pleasing to the eye, emanates from that center. Here is Sita's testimonial after an East Indian dance performed on three consecutive nights:

"I felt a lot of anxiety before dancing. I didn't know the right thing to do in order to help myself stay centered, so I started taking Almond a week before the performances. It was an incredible experience how much it helped me, first to be focused on everything that I did. I saw that I was doing everything I needed to do, but not from an emotional state—more coming from my spine. This helped me to feel what it is like to be 'in the spine.' The day of the first performance, I was very centered. I didn't have any anxiety. I was even surprised—the last time I'd had so much fear. My hands and feet had been very cold, and I had stomach pains. Taking Almond is like a magician giving you something. Every time I took it, it transformed me. Almond helped me to do a perfect job, a perfect performance."

NEGATIVE INDICATIONS

The negative Almond state is that spread-too-thin feeling, as though there is never enough time. When no matter how much we accomplish we can't quite get the job done, it is time for Almond. Tension typically sets off a predictable chain reaction of progressively less productivity that can backslide into a state of complete frustration. Almond, through the quality of calmness, allows us to focus on one thing at a time—and before long a whole stack of incoming work has moved into the outgoing file!

As previously mentioned, Almond also addresses the issue of

human sexuality. When the loud hormones of adolescence speak, and any time thereafter when sexual energy seems uncontrollable, Almond may be of benefit. (Please note that Almond falls in the Spectrum's third Quadrant of drive tempered by self-control, rather than in the second Quadrant of fiery youth where it would not yet have reached a deeper maturity.) One study after another reveals that adolescents in the United States are having intercourse at earlier ages than ever before. Sexually transmitted diseases, some with death as a contraindication, run rampant. The federal centers for Disease Control and Prevention have documented a rise in AIDS cases from 49,016 in 1992 to 103,500 in 1993—a 111 percent increase. The issue of sexuality in our era covers the entire gamut from creating to destroying human life.

Consider, too, the exploitation of this powerful drive through the media. Even ads for items as innocuous as soda pop are unmistakably sexually charged. Constantly bombarded both visually and aurally, what are we to do? Add to this phenomena a diet fully loaded with preservatives, pesticides, and artificial stimulants that play havoc with the sex nerves, and it is clear that we are being overstimulated and encouraged in the direction of excess. Almond is a healthy counter-attack to these detrimental outer stimuli.

No, Almond does not weaken, repress or annihilate sexual energy; rather, it allows us to transmute this powerful force. With this essence, one might say that instead of being driven by our sex drive, we become the driver, through consciously exercising self-control. Sexual energy being our creative force, we might choose to reroute that energy into athletics or creative pursuits, such as painting or the performing arts. Whether in a relationship or single, young or old, Almond provides us with a deeper understanding of sexuality as pure energy at our disposal.

THEME CHARACTERISTICS

Almond themes are not as easily detected through physical clues as other themes because their energy flows inward and upward rather than out through their senses and physical body. Their movements are neither grand nor small; their pace is neither too fast nor too slow. In other words, they are conspicuously inconspicuous! They do not stand out in a crowd like Pineapple or off to the side like Banana. Neither wallflowers nor party animals, you probably won't even find them at social gatherings. They are neither social nor antisocial. The lifestyles of monks, nuns, hermits, and ascetics fit comfortably for the inwardly focused Almond theme.

As a rule, Almond themes don't take second helpings—except to honor their hostess. And, like Goldilocks, they prefer their porridge not too hot or too cold, but just right. These are quiet, interiorized people who use their time and energy wisely. One feels their magnetism of calmness born of moderate, balanced living. Almond themes inspire us to put our own lives in order, simply by their example of how well an orderly life works.

FAMOUS THEME PERSONALITIES

Omar Khayyam
Ralph Waldo Emerson
Goldilocks
Buddha
Ableza in "Hanta Yo"
St. Anthony of the Desert
Nijinsky
Rabi'a
Thomas á Kempis

Omar Khayyam, the son of a tent-maker (also the meaning of his last name), was an eleventh-century Persian astronomer, mathematician, and poet. That little is known of his personal life is compensated for by the richness of his quatrains comprising "The Rubaiyat," one of the best known and loved poems of all times. This Almond theme's deep spiritual message pours through the wisdom of his writing.

Misunderstood as a hedonist glorifying sensual excess—or one chronically stuck in the negative Almond state—Omar's poetry reveals him as a great mystic. (His quatrains have been interpreted by Yogananda in a stunning rendition listed in the bibliography.) In the purest of verse, Omar exhorts us to channel our energy inward, away from all overindulgence, to the highest possible attainment. His words are an Almond theme's admonition to totally redirect our life force away from the senses and into the astral spine. The deepest and only lasting joy, he tells us, is found in the wine of Spirit, not in the false intoxicants of sensual pursuits.

CONFESSIONS OF AN ALMOND THEME: THOM SHARES

"I am absolutely dedicated to making this lifetime all it can be in all directions. That's a balancing act. I am in a stage of actively building my business from scratch. I sell personal growth seminars. My work is play right now. Nothing I do is work, and I totally love it. So my energy's flowing. I love what I'm doing, and I pretty much go flat out with it.

"I enjoy meeting people. But I have to have appreciable time alone in my own space. Spare time? I have none. I always have ideas. It is a continual battle for me to prioritize and separate the wheat from the chaff. My girlfriend helps me with balance. On Sundays we go for walks in pretty places, or go to a movie or something like that.

"My spiritual practices have changed me a lot. I used to have pretty high sexual energy. Now that I'm over fifty. . . whatever. My girlfriend and I will make love every once in a great while when she would like it for a feeling of closeness and bonding. For me now, it has nothing to do with my gratification. Self-control is really important to me. All I can say is that I'm healthier and stronger, and I've got more energy than ever in my life.

"Yes, I would say I'm a calm person. I'm pretty unruffled. I like to think I'm close to the way Napoleon was, sitting in the battlefield writing a letter when a cannonball landed right beside him. He used the sand from the cannonball to dry the ink on his letter. I don't know where I heard that story, but it was given to me as the epitome of calmness.

"I do like almonds. When I'm organized enough, every day of my life I carry almonds around as part of my afternoon snack with fruit. I definitely like almonds, though I don't eat them every day. I think they're the quintessential food."

WRAPPING IT UP

Some years ago, I found myself—somewhat by accident, I might add—on a large pleasure-cruise ocean liner routed from Southern California to several Mexican ports. During our first-night orientation program, the social director encouraged—or rather exhorted—us to eat and drink to excess, gamble and carouse all night, and wear ourselves out as if there were no tomorrow. To our privileged group was revealed the unwritten Eleventh Commandment: Thou shalt not count calories. The message behind all this fanfare was that excessive behavior—or "letting ourselves go"—would deepen our happiness and enrich our vacation experience. And besides, what are holidays for anyway?

As the English poet John Milton intuited, "He who reigns within himself, and rules passions, desires and fears, is more than a king." True happiness lies in balance; fulfillment, tempered by self-respect, is found in moderation. Our passion for life, expressed through moral vigor, need not deplete us. Indeed, we can be strengthened by it. The zeal of this essence can help us tap into vast reserves of calmness. By transforming ourselves, we can inspire others as well.

ALMOND	Contrasted With:	Companioned With:
Banana	for calmness through non-identification with the ego	for the wisdom to discriminate beyond the level of emotions and desires
Fig	for wisdom through willingness to look at all of an issue	for flexibility, not laxity; a soft approach while holding firm to healthful ideals
Lettuce	for calmness and clarity with emotion and feeling, respectively	for being centered in oneself and respectful of what is needed to stay in balance
Spinach	for stress due to over-work living too much in one's head	for a tension-free, fun-loving attitude
Tomato	for acknowledging, and completely eliminating, addictions	for mental and emotional health and strength in battling excesses and addictions

POSITIVE EXPRESSIONS

Moderate

Balanced

Efficient

Temperance-seeking

Avoiding harmful substances

Calm

Sexually well-adjusted

Inward by nature

Self-controlled

Sensitive partner in relationship

Disciplined

Quiet

Silence-loving

Interiorized

NEGATIVE CONDITIONS

Nervous	Discontent
Excessiveness-prone	Uneasy
Lacking in control	Stressed
Rebellious	Never caught up
Addictive in personality	Frustrated
Sexually immoderate	"Workaholic"-prone
Habit-bound	Restless

ESSENCE ENHANCERS

Allow more time than needed to finish projects in order to avoid feeling rushed by deadlines.

Give yourself a five-minute neck and shoulder rub, finishing with a full minute on your scalp—or enlist the help of a friend.

Do the following breathing exercise three times in succession, three times a day: inhale with two quick inhalations, the second deeper than the first, until the lungs are completely filled. Exhale in the same way: twice strongly, until the lungs are fully emptied.

Spend a full day or longer in complete silence without speaking. Observe the changes in your energy flow from this practice. When nerves in the tongue are activated through movement, restlessness is created in the brain.

Go dancing, dance in your home, or enroll in a dance class. Become aware of the energy in your spine through practicing this art form and consciously direct it inward and upward.

Repeat the Almond visualization daily.

VISUALIZATION

It is a perfect day for a short walk and your third day on vacation. The worries and responsibilities of work, home, and family all seem dreamlike now, as though they belonged to someone else. Breathe in the fresh morning air as you leave your little cabin in the woods and walk toward the creek bed. Nighttime, you notice, has receded, lifting itself layer by quilted layer, off the earth's shoulders. An Indian summer day, it is already warm and promising to grow hotter.

A thick scattering of bright orange poppies blankets the field. Drink in this color through your eyes, your hands, and the pores of your skin. Feel it warming you, healing you, and bathing your cells in a pure ray of orange light.

Continuing on your walk, you approach a swirl of fallen tree limbs covered with moss. Take off your sandals and run your toes through the velvet greenery. Now, sit near the creek where the water splashes over rocks and crags. Breathe this sound into your ears, your lung, and every cell in your body. Allow it to wash away all tension, leaving a flowing stream of calmness in its wake. Replace any thoughts of excess with moderation; any overindulgences with self-control.

Having bathed your senses in the pure orange light, consciously withdraw from them—first from sight, then sound, followed by taste, touch, and scent. Imagine that you are retreating into the core of your being You are being recharged, renewed, and reawakened in the vast store-house of energy that is your truest reality.

AFFIRMATION

I am the master of my destiny! With calm power I stride toward the horizon to final victory!

CHAPTER TWENTY-ONE

PEAR:
"THE PEACEMAKER"

Pyrus communis
("the common pear")

"I was feeling really anxious before starting on Pear. Now I'm more relaxed and don't feel like I have to do everything right this moment. Lately, I've decided to work on my relationship with my mother, so I started the Pear three days before Thanksgiving. Finally after thirty-four years, I was able to talk to her. The blocks dissolved. Mom opened up too. You could say Pear triggered a clearing of the air between us."

—*EH, Seattle, WA*

"Pear is definitely helping me. I must admit that I've not been very regular in taking it. But this past week in particular I have acted much more from a place of inner peacefulness despite a most hectic and demanding schedule at the clinic."   —*SLP, North San Juan, CA*

"Last week I was awakened at 4:30 a.m. by a vehicle down the street that exploded into flames. Needless to say, my heart was pounding! Pear helped me get through this disturbance, and to regain composure and calm down enough to meditate—even while the fire engine was still on the street with the motor running and lights flashing."

—*LF, Taos, NM*

"My husband and I took a two-day trip, leaving our twenty-one-month-old son with people he likes. I gave him Pear for the emotional trauma of us being gone. He did well—didn't nap as much and still woke up happy, not cranky. He is also learning to walk now and falls down a lot, so Pear is helping here as well."   —*LB, Nevada City, CA*

"After the last big earthquake in Los Angeles, I felt really drawn to eating pears, which is unusual for me. Well, I can take a hint—I'm about to start taking Pear Essence!"   —*NL, Los Angeles, CA*

"Peace gave us the seasons.
Peace gave us the rain,
Cool clouds that gather to bless us,
Mist hands that soothe away pain." —I. Donald Walters

FLOWER/FRUIT/FOLKLORE

Pears are native to Western Asia and Europe and grow in all temperate regions. Their date of origin is unknown, though the Greek poet Homer mentioned them in his writings in the 700's B.C. Pear trees are hardy and grow in almost any type of soil. The flower—a delicate, full-petaled white in color—is cross-pollinated and grows in clusters of four to twelve blossoms. Pear varieties number in the hundreds. Pears are significantly high in vitamin C and iron. They are an excellent digestive aid and, due to their delicate mineral balance, a fine complexion toner.

Quality: Peacefulness, Emergency Essence
Message of Self-mastery: Peace of mind; returns a sense of rhythm and proportion; for being fully in the present moment; ability to handle crisis; for stability during major changes.
Pattern of Disharmony: Feeling thrown off balance during accidents, illness, surgery or childbirth; physical and/or emotional crisis; auric disturbances, minor to monumental; for shock, or thought or fear of it; extreme grief; for any troubling experience.

SPECTRUM PLACEMENT

Emerging from the calmness of Almond, we find Pear in Quadrant III's second house. This remedy has an unmistakable, unshakable strength. Pear's is the pure strength of being totally centered, completely balanced, and absolutely in control of our faculties— all valuable assets in the face of emergency situations. With its own masculine-tinted "take charge" energy, it emits Quadrant III's experienced know-how. If the tranquility of Almond is the calm before the storm, then Pear is the peace after it.

POSITIVE APPLICATIONS

Webster's dictionary defines peace as "freedom from war or civil strife, an agreement to end war." Indeed, the positive Pear state is exactly that—the resolution of war, or conflict, within ourselves. Peace, like calmness, is often mistaken for a state of low energy, sinking at times to the level of boredom. Nothing happening, nothing to do—hmm, must be peace. But true peace is quite the opposite. It's that state of victory in which battles are fought and won; when great challenges are accepted and not shunned; where we come face to face with the enemy in conflict and say, "Leave: now." These battles may take the physical form of accidents, surgeries, or major illnesses. Such events, when viewed from a superconscious level, need not be interpreted as negative experiences; rather, they are opportunities for growth. Pear is our Emergency Essence. (Take it more often during crisis and apply it directly to the skin if desired.)

Or, the challenge may be that of childbirth in which Pear's positive qualities are invaluable. Some years ago, a woman who had chosen to deliver at home suffered a hypoglycemic attack during transition. Her husband administered Pear every five minutes and within half an hour, she had stopped shaking and was able to continue with the birth. Pear is especially helpful for the first-time mother who is taken by surprise to learn that the word "labor" is a gross understatement of the experience. Here, she reasons that childbirth falls into the category of an ill-timed dental appointment from which she can, by choice, simply walk away and reschedule at her convenience. (I remember asking my brother, an osteopath, if his wife was going to deliver their first-born by natural childbirth. "Are you kidding?" he looked at me, astonished. "To Patty, that means with no make-up.") At that point when a woman wants to turn back, deciding that she's "had enough, thank you," Pear acts as a "vibrational midwife," offering peace and comfort. In other words, Pear can help the mother, and those who assist her, to experience the transcendent nature of birth.

The positive Pear state also expresses willingness and openness to face the unknown. As Ashley wrote, "I had tried skiing years ago and was terrified. I tried once more recently, and my boyfriend said he'd never seen anyone do so well the first time."

Pear is strengthening to the aura. A bad case of nerves, depression, fear, or trauma all weaken this protective layer of energy around the body, leaving us vulnerable to further aftershocks from emotional earthquakes. "Today in particular," wrote Frances, "I was very nervous before I met some customers to write an offer to buy a condominium. I felt insecure and thought that they might think I was too young or didn't know enough of real estate. So I took Pear because I was starting to lose control. I was almost shaking. Toward the middle of the transaction, I was starting to feel very confident about my knowledge and how I was presenting myself to them. It all worked out fine, and I closed a very large sale."

"I have Chronic Fatigue Syndrome, which is why I had to retire from a wonderful editorial career," Syd shared. "For the last seven years, Christmas has been a profoundly depressing time for me. I felt total despair as I watched my body getting worse and worse. I was a prisoner—oppressed and unable to pull myself out of despondency. On Pear, I experienced an immediate change of attitude: peace and hope. There are no physical changes—just a one-hundred-eighty-degree turnaround emotionally. Every day on Pear is a revelation, and I just had a very happy Christmas!"

NEGATIVE INDICATIONS

And what exactly are the circumstances that rob us of our peace? Conflict, for one; resistance, for another. When in conflict, we are in the negative Pear state meaning, simply, the absence of peace. Interpersonal relationships—those flawless mirrors of our strengths and weaknesses alike—offer the perfect setting for Pear. "I felt the consciousness of peace come into my body with the first drop of Pear," Melissa commented. "My husband got upset with me, but I was able to stay calm."

When avoidance of conflict masquerades as peace, we find repression instead, one of the great destroyers of true peace of mind. When family conflicts remain buried for months or even decades, Pear can be a much needed catalyst in building healthy relationships.

Let's talk now about resistance. Purely in terms of energy flows, when we resist the tests that life gives us, pain can be the end result. Fighting *against* inevitable tests only creates blocks. Just giving in, on the other hand, errs in the opposite direction of passivity, which implies a lack of energy and thus no magnetism to draw the answers we need. Dylan Thomas' famous poem, "Do Not Go Gentle Into That Good Night," comes to mind. Written for his dying father, Thomas implores him to "rage, rage, against the dying of the light." It's fine to exit this world in a blaze of light, alive and joyful to the last. But to rage against what is trying to happen is the resistance of which we are speaking, the kind that only inhibits and disrupts the natural flow of events. It's Pear, the peacemaker to the rescue.

THEME CHARACTERISTICS

Pear themes have a distinctly powerful energy. Why? Because they are at peace with themselves. You will often find them in the healing professions, similar to Raspberry themes. It matters not if they are massage therapists, Rolfers, flower remedy practitioners, or allopathic personnel; even being near them is much like receiving a treatment.

Their body language is fluid but definite in a paradox of stillness in motion. The more developed their Pear-like qualities, the more pronounced the paradox. Mentally, Pear themes are even-tempered and not easily ruffled. Their fluid nature allows conflict to roll off them like water off the proverbial duck's back.

Here's an interesting sidelight about Pear themes—their homes are unusually homey and inviting. A healing vibration pervades. You'll feel like overstaying your welcome, no matter what the architecture or interior design—and will be looking for excuses to stay longer!

One senses in their magnetism the harmony of the seasons—the cycles of night following day, much like resolution in the wake of friction. These are people who "walk their talk." For this reason, Pear themes exemplify the connectedness to the earth of the Native Americans. They make fascinating armchair philosophers and possess an earthy sense of humor. Be prepared—you'll find yourself wanting to "just hang around" them, absorbing their peacefulness like a squirrel gathering nuts for wintertime.

FAMOUS THEME PERSONALITIES

Dwight D. Eisenhower
John Adams
Christian Slater
Andie McDowell
Michael Jordan
King Arthur
Simba's father in "The Lion King"
James Earl Jones
Hippocrates

"I like Ike" became the motto for our thirty-fourth president. Dwight Eisenhower was, without question, a peaceable, and peace-loving man. Ike, who served in both World Wars, is best described as a man of democratic simplicity and outgoing warmth. Although he was not the best military strategist, people felt his keen leadership abilities. Rich in the Pear qualities of caution and reconciliation, Ike accepted the surrender of the Germans in 1945; initiated a truce in 1953 which ended the Korean war; temporarily relaxed USSR tensions in 1955 at his meeting with Khrushchev; and negotiated a peaceful end to the Suez crisis. This peace-seeking president demonstrated Pear's theme qualities to a monumental degree, magnetizing an end to war on a global level many times over.

His written words too are permeated with a potent vibration of peacefulness. Personally indifferent to the civil rights of blacks, he nonetheless used federal troops to desegregate schools in Atlanta in 1955. "I am deeply sympathetic," he commiserated, "with the efforts of any group to enjoy the rights of equality that they are guaranteed by the Constitution." Eisenhower, in both speech and deed, emulates the steadfastness, balance, and harmony of a true Pear theme.

CONFESSIONS OF A PEAR THEME: JERRY SPEAKS

"I'm property manager of an apartment complex. For years and years, I was a steel contractor. I think I'm very Taurean. I'm down-to-earth practical, I like things to work smoothly. I wouldn't consider myself very creative. I'm more of a worker bee than someone who thinks up new projects. Manager is a good position for me. I tend to be conservative. I like to have projects to work on.

"It's uncomfortable for me to be around people with real highs and real lows. I like nice and steady energy. I feel real uneasy and awkward around people who fly off the handle, and then I'm always on eggshells around them because I don't know when they'll fly off again. On one hand, I feel compassion for them. I think I have to work on being with people like that. You have difficulty being around things that touch nerves in you.

"I generally consider myself a peaceful person. It's very important to me—harmony, keeping the peace. In any situation, I don't mind compromising. I really don't like disharmony. Even if it's going toward something better, it eats away at me. So I'm always willing to try to work it out, let it go, and then not worry about it. One thing I could probably work on is knowing when to compromise and when not to. You know, when it's a matter of principle, you can give away too much, and you lose some integrity. But I love to keep the peace and harmony, and try to get sides to just come together. Someone said I'm a good diplomat. I can't stand unrest. It's a difficult thing, knowing when to fight and when to say, 'Well, it's not that big a deal.'

"I don't freak out in an emergency. People tell me, 'Oh, you look so calm up there,' when I have to give a talk. My dad was like that too. No matter what would happen, he was unflappable. So, yeah, I try to be calm like that and not get freaked out. I just always want to restore things back to order—as long as it doesn't get boring. See, you run the risk of boring people around you to death, always trying to stop any conflict before it starts.

"Pears? I do like pears. It's hard to find good ones. They're picked so unripe these days that by the time they get to market, why bother?

When we were in Italy, my wife and I ate some fruit called apple pears. They were the most amazing fruit we've ever had in our lives. They were just the perfect ripeness, you know?"

Wrapping It Up

The true message of Pear is to remain untouched by the passing tragedies and tremors of life. Ancient yogic teachings remind us that every outward joy is followed by pain, and every pain by a period of joy. When we live in this realization, we become pillars of strength and comfort to those in need.

By now, you get the picture. Peace is not the result of passivity. The "pearl of great price"—peace—is rarely, if ever, handed to us on a platter. Peace, to the contrary, is the hard-earned result of great effort and thus, greatness. For this reason we may rightly consider Pear to be the sum total of all the positive traits of all twenty Spirit-in-Nature Essences: perfect peace, perfect calmness, perfect love. The tiny drops of Pear are indeed "the mist hands that soothe away pain."

PEAR	Contrasted With:	Companioned With:
Coconut	sticking with challenges	perseverance through especially difficult tests, including emergencies
Grape	wholeness through giving love	for an upward flow of dependable energy; strong, unwavering love
Lettuce	calmness due to quieted emotions	to enhance the quality calmness on deeper levels
Tomato	for fighting battles	for calm courage and great stamina

POSITIVE EXPRESSIONS

Peaceful

Composed

Living in the present

Earthy

Balanced

Conflict-resolving

Strong

Open

Willing

A peacemaker

Solid

Fluid

Harmonious

Loving

Cautious

Reconciliatory

Centered

Compromising

Steady

NEGATIVE CONDITIONS

Traumatized

Nervous

Unresolved in conflict

Unbalanced in emergencies

Tense

Resistant

Friction-prone

Unresolved in relationships

Experiencing auric disturbances

Shock-prone

Experiencing extreme grief

Vulnerable

Feeling "out of sorts"

Brash

Hasty

Quarrelsome

Uncentered

ESSENCE ENHANCERS

Take a first aid and/or CPR course; learn to handle crisis situations. Visit friends and relatives in hospitals and nursing homes.

Watch an occasional film that depicts a strong element of conflict. Learn to view life as a passing dream.

Go for long walks in the country or at the oceanside. Consciously tune in to the natural rhythms of the trees, the wind, and the waves.

VISUALIZATION

Although you have just arrived at the lakeshore, it seems that you have been here a long, long time. Perhaps each of the seasons has brushed against your sleeve as you sat here. You know there have not been any waves, or your feet would be soaked to the bone by now.

Remember how, as a child, you used to skip flat stones on the water's surface, counting how many times they danced before sinking? Pick up the nearest pebble, worn smooth by the relentless washing of the water. With a deft flick of your wrist, send it on its way. Good. Got the feel of it?

Now send several more stones across the lake's smooth surface. Imagine each of them to be a particular conflict or a point of unrest in your life. As they sink one by one to their watery grave, allow a sense of resolution and inner peace to steal into your being. All is resolved. All is harmoniously balanced.

AFFIRMATION

Smilingly I greet life's difficulties, seeing all of them as gay flowers in a meadow that nod with encouragement and opportunity.

CHAPTER TWENTY-TWO

AVOCADO:
"THE MINDFUL ONE"

Persea americana
("American alligator pear")

"Avocado helped me with focus and clarity of thought, despite a diagnosed chemical imbalance in my brain."   —*HJ, Downey, CA*

"I took Avocado because I needed to carry through with the details of a project. Now I've written out a 'to do' list that really helps me stay organized."   —*RJ, Ontario, Canada*

"Avocado has helped my memory. I am able to live more in the present but can also recall and retain past events much easier than before. I also remember my dreams in greater detail when I take Avocado right before. I go to sleep."   —*MR, London, England*

"My friend said she got an A on her midterm after taking Avocado."   —*TS, Mountain View, CA*

"I cook at a retreat center. My week on Avocado produced very creative dishes. Because I'm also an artist, I felt I could bring all my talents together into the cooking: balancing color, new ways of doing grains and vegetables. Every day, I was amazed."   —*BA, North San Juan, CA*

"I've been at an emotional crossroads with my husband. Avocado has helped me to feel more guidance and direction."   —*ML, Rocklin, CA*

"Lull'd in the countless chambers of the brain,
Our thoughts are link'd by many a hidden chain;
Awake but one, and lo, what myriads rise!
Each stamps its image as the other flies." —Alexander Pope

FLOWER/FRUIT/FOLKLORE

Aztec priests attributed aphrodisiac powers to this luscious fruit native to central America that now grows in subtropical areas such as Florida and California. An evergreen of the laurel family, the tree reaches a height of sixty feet. The avocado pear is propagated by the seed. Its flowers, small and white, grow in terminal clusters. There are over four hundred varieties of avocados, ranging in size and color. The avocado, called a perfect food for its balance and abundance of nutrients, is high in calories and fat (twenty-five percent) from it's fruit oil content. Rich in fourteen essential minerals, vitamin B, and protein, it helps to regulate bodily functions and stimulate growth. Helping to lower blood cholesterol, relieving psoriasis, and toning the skin and hair are some of its medicinal properties.

Quality: Good memory
Message of Self-mastery: Mental focus; remembering details; joy in challenging the mind; for exams, puzzles, word games; new projects; greater awareness; attitude of *"now* I get it"; for tracing back to past traumas with clarity; helps past issues to surface to the conscious mind; learning from mistakes.
Pattern of Disharmony: Forgetfulness; absent-mindedness; dullness; missing details; going along without purpose or direction; for the "out to lunch" state; "sowing wild oats."

SPECTRUM PLACEMENT

With Pear planting us firmly on the ground, we now move to Quadrant III's third house—Avocado. From Pear's steadiness arises the clarity and sharp mental focus of Avocado. This essence contains

Quadrant III's maturity and the Spectrum's masculine virtues of manifested strength through the joy of mental challenges. In no uncertain terms, Avocado represents a solid mental footing—knowing ourselves and the direction we want to take with our lives.

POSITIVE APPLICATIONS

The positive Avocado state is like opening a window in a boarded-up room. Avocado not only awakens attentiveness, but the zeal to apply ourselves as well. Instead of being mentally absent, day-dreamy, disorganized and spacey, we are awake and alert. Avocado boasts that state of readiness to complete the task before us, be it studying for an exam or making a major career decision. Positive Avocado implies a strong sense of direction and the willingness to move forward with clear intention.

The following story humorously illustrates Avocado's mental focus and fixity of purpose:

"My son is a football player," wrote Colleen. "In his first year at college he was told by a professor, 'Buddy, keep going the way you are, and you'll be out of here soon. You're digging yourself in deep.'

"He was in college only for football," she continued, "wondering in his freshman year how he was going to get through four years of university. On a hunch, I put him on Avocado. All of a sudden, he was studying and bringing his homework to breakfast. My 210-pound, 6'4" son had developed a love for French, history, and literature!"

Avocado's message of good memory extends beyond shopping lists and the ability to tag correct names onto long-forgotten faces. Its motto is mental dexterity—a mind poised at the starting gate, waiting to begin the race; an intellect that welcomes unsolvable problems and mental endurance tests, much like a well-toned athlete looking forward to training sessions. The mind is like a muscle; the more we exercise it, the more it grows.

NEGATIVE INDICATIONS

Conversely, the negative Avocado state manifests as attitudes of shirking and shrinking. These noncommittal mindsets—always self-chosen—leave us on the sidelines, rendering us spectators of our own lives. In the negative Avocado state, we repeat the same mistakes over and over because we "just don't get it." I have a friend who jokingly says that he always makes different mistakes, thus refusing to succumb to the negative Avocado state. What he is actually saying is that he is at least putting out the energy to learn from his mistakes, thereby eliminating the need to repeat them.

Being dreamy, forgetful, and anywhere but in the moment indicate the need for Avocado. Living in the past is another negative Avocado trait. So is regretting past words or actions we cannot change. Avocado deals with the *quality* of our thoughts, both waking and sleeping. Many people report changes in their dreams on Avocado. When the conscious mind is sharpened, the subconscious mind may then also reflect a certain clarity.

THEME CHARACTERISTICS

Avocado themes and those in the positive Avocado state love to ask questions, fix things, figure out how they work, and why they don't. Doing something in a new way is thrilling for them. Designing, solving and studying are favorite pastimes of the Avocado theme. There's no mental couch potato here! In fact, the stereotypical computer nerd could well be an Avocado theme. One important distinction between Avocado and Corn themes is that Avocados are the *mental* explorers of an intellectual wilderness, while Corn themes pioneer the land and sea through their *physical* actions.

These themes express a strong energy characteristic of Quadrant III. Avocado theme women possess a well developed masculine nature. And both the men and women will have a strong sense of identity, purpose and direction. Visually oriented, they often have intense eyes and look directly into yours when speaking to you, just as they look intensely into the nature of things. They are alert and focused. Their magnetism draws others out of any mental sloppiness, their energy wordlessly admonishing, "Wake up!"

FAMOUS THEME PERSONALITIES

Stephen Hawking
Bobby Fischer
Bill Gates
Data of "Star Trek"
Dr. Spock of "Star Trek"
Walt Disney
Stephen Spielberg
Carl Jung
Admiral Richard Byrd
Sherlock Holmes

Only an Avocado theme would even attempt to solve the puzzles and paradoxes of the universe. Born in 1942 on the anniversary of Galileo's death, Stephen William Hawking is considered one of the great minds of this century—and is one of few overqualified for his position as an Avocado theme! This British theoretical physicist, in true Avocado form, sought to explain the mysteries of deep space, black holes, and the Big Bang theory.

Professor Hawking now speaks through a voice synthesizer. He has been confined to a wheel chair since 1966 when he was diagnosed with Lou Gehrig's disease, an incurable degenerative disorder of the nervous system. A Coconut sub-theme, he has tackled the most challenging physical tests and turned them to his advantage. Only without the distracting influences of a functional body, he affirms, can he have the mental freedom for his work.

Carl Sagan writes in the introduction to the professor's ground breaking book, A Brief History Of Time: "Hawking is attempting, as he explicitly states, to understand the mind of God. And this makes all the more unexpected the conclusion of the effort, at least so far: a universe with no edge in space, no beginning or end in time, and nothing for a Creator to do."

CONFESSIONS OF AN AVOCADO THEME: IN BRUCE'S WORDS

"Quirks to my personality? I love change, and I tend to set up routines for myself—which is a paradox. I get the most fun out of concentrating on doing one thing, and yet most of the time I'm doing many things at once. Sometimes it's the nature of my work. My mind is easily sidetracked into doing other things. I'm a jack of all trades, so to speak, and an administrator of a retreat facility.

"My mind is extremely active but very much out of control most of the time. It loves humor. I just love to laugh. Emotions—well, I got lots of 'em! When I actually get down to dealing with them as opposed to just being swamped by them, I'm not really into the psychological approach to things. I'm after deeper change than that—like affirmations.

"I tend to be quiet in a group situation. I would rather listen than talk. I enjoy listening, so it's not like I'm stuffing it or anything. To make a long story short, other people are more interesting to me than I am. I tend to make very different kinds of friends—people who would not be friends with one another. Like in school, I was friends with the jocks, with the dopers, with people who studied hard, and friends with people who partied. I attribute this to feeling that I don't need people to validate my behavior in order for them to be worth knowing. I don't feel that somebody has to be doing what I'm doing with my life to be an interesting, enjoyable person. It's just the stimulation of hearing about different experiences and different ways of looking at things.

"I definitely have a learning desire—for experience even more than learning. I like to know about things, but I don't like to go through the process of learning. But experiences—I just enjoy different experiences. I have a good memory, not a tremendous memory. I remember people, tend to be able to remember things I've read, even down to where it was on the page. Not photographic, though. The mental side of my nature is dominant, it's happening.

"I love avocados, they're one of my favorites. Well, my family used to have an avocado grove. It was a beautiful place to work—I loved working there in about ten acres of avocado trees. I had almost no experience with them until I was about sixteen and then, since we had the grove, I figured I should taste them. I couldn't really tune in to them very well—they're an acquired taste. Now I think they're really wonderful. I like them in sandwiches, in salads, in omelettes, or alone with a touch of tamari. To me, you just don't put avocados together with oranges. They don't belong with fruits, even though they are one."

WRAPPING IT UP

Some years ago I enrolled in a calligraphy class taught by a very lively older man—and a perfect Avocado theme. As a grand finale to the last class, he recited by heart several long and melodious poems by a currently fashionable author. "They say if you can memorize," he added, "you can retain your memory longer." Indeed, memory loss is not an occupational hazard of the aging process. A weak memory, Paramhansa Yogananda advised us, is caused by two things: lack of concentration; and the mental blocks people raise in rejection against some of life's experiences.

The Sanskrit word *smriti*, meaning remembrance of our true state of perfection, is an apt definition for Avocado. Indeed, we have nothing, or "no thing," to learn—we need only remember. Oscar Wilde defines memory as "the diary that we all carry about with us." This diary is our autobiography, carved out of our unique lessons—trials, errors, and all—as well as the memory of who we truly are. Avocado helps us to be consciously aware that the moment we mold in the present moment is our opportunity to remember our own perfection.

AVOCADO	*Contrasted With:*	*Companioned With:*
Corn	for a more general flow of energy	for clarity and focused energy
Fig	for attention to detail	for seeing the bigger picture as well as details
Orange	for enthusiasm	for remembering that joy is our true nature

POSITIVE EXPRESSIONS

Willing	Attentive to detail
Open	Lucid dreaming
Good memory retention	Strongly directional
Mindful	Purposeful
Aware	Able to learn lessons
Alert	Organized
Accurate	Clear thinking
Acuity-oriented	Living fully in the present
Mentally ready	Able to concentrate

NEGATIVE CONDITIONS

Forgetful	Spacey
Noncommittal	Vacant-minded
Day-dreamy	Absent-minded
Regretful	Dull
Sloppy	Inattentive to detail
Repeating mistakes	Unambitious
Holding onto the past	Unconscious
Disorganized	Homesick

ESSENCE ENHANCERS

Mentally challenge yourself with word games, board games, and puzzles.

Learn a foreign language and plan a trip to a country where it is spoken.

Invent something—mechanical, culinary, or whatever sparks your imagination—and test it out.

Take a night class or correspondence course in an area of interest.

At bedtime, mentally review the events of the day and what you have learned from them.

VISUALIZATION

It is the peak of autumn. The cloak of a cooler climate envelops the ground. The misty October winds entice the clouds to clap with thunderous delight, applauding the chilly afternoon. Droplets of rain trickle through the heavens' upturned palms. Amorphous pools of water collect in the rutted gravel road beneath your feet. If you don't step carefully around them, your walking shoes will soon be soaked.

Remember being a child and stepping smack in the middle of the puddles—directly after being told not to? Well, no one's looking—go ahead. Splash and stir as loudly as you like. Now, step back and squat down beside the puddle. Once clear, now it is clouded. How like a distracted, unfocused mind, this mud puddle! The crystal raindrops of moments ago are now a "sedimental mess."

Focus on this little pool of water. Watch what happens as the mud of directionless, distracted thoughts settles. Clarity returns. Purpose and mindfulness surface once again.

Call up this image, like a file on your mental computer, whenever your mind is clouded. Transmute the erstwhile muddle of forgetfulness into the crystal pool of remembrance.

AFFIRMATION

I accept willingly all that comes to me, for all things are divine gifts of love!

CHAPTER TWENTY-THREE

APPLE:

"THE CLEAR

MENTAL SKIES"

Pyrus malus
("apple, pear, or crab apple:
a fleshy exterior fruit")

"I asked myself, 'What do I need?' and my brain said, 'Apple.' And I started taking it and I felt better."   —*RG, Nevada City, CA*

"I had major colon surgery nine days ago. For the last week, I have been craving apples. This is very strange because apples are not one of my favorite fruits, and I don't usually seek them out. I take this as a sign to start on Apple."   —*EH, North San Juan, CA*

"Even though I can hardly tolerate apples due to the sugar content, my kinesiologist found Apple to be strengthening to a number of my organs. We were both amazed!"   —*JP, Oklahoma City, OK*

"Apple has backed up the clarity of my mind with physical vitality. I've had the energy from 6:30 to 9 in the evening to do the programs here. I wouldn't have done it before."

—*EA Nevada City, CA*

"I was feeling groggy and took Apple. My wife said I was totally different afterwards—and friendlier!"   —*RM, Fort Worth, TX*

*"The surest road to health, say what they will, is never
to suppose we shall be ill."*   —Churchill

FLOWER/FRUIT/FOLKLORE

Apples, members of the rose family, are the most widely cultivated
fruit of temperate regions. Rich in folklore since the biblical Garden
of Eden, they date back at least three thousand years. Apples were also
described in the hieroglyphic writings discovered in ancient Egyptian
pyramids and tombs. There are at least six thousand varieties of apples.
The clustered blossoms on leafy stems may be white, pink, or rose,
depending upon the variety. Apples contain about fifty percent more
vitamin C than oranges and a significant amount of the rare vitamin G,
"the appetite vitamin," that promotes growth and digestion. As powerful blood purifiers, apples benefit the lymphatic system, intestines,
and arteries. They also lower blood pressure and reduce tooth decay.

Quality: Peaceful Clarity
Message of Self-mastery: Mental clarity; healthy, magnetic attitudes;
an abundance of psychologically nourishing thoughts; hope; motiva-
tion to take better care of oneself; a positive outlook.
Pattern of Disharmony: mental fuzziness; health-related fears; worry;
doubt; indecision; recurrence of toxic emotions such as anger, jealousy,
and fear; a sense of physical or emotional vulnerability.

SPECTRUM PLACEMENT

From the clarity of Avocado, we enter Quadrant III's fourth house,
to Apple. Avocado's keen memory leads to Apple's acuity. The old folk
remedy, "an apple a day keeps the doctor away," has a ring of truth to
it. Overflowing with this Quadrant's crisp strength and "harvestabil-
ity," Apple lays the groundwork for the zest of Orange, its successor.
Through Apple, we come to a wonderful understanding of the subtle
dance between the body, mind, and spirit. When these elements are
harmonized, the result is a state of radiant well-being.

POSITIVE APPLICATIONS

Apple Essence doesn't heal physical symptoms, as explained in an earlier chapter. It does, however, aid in stimulating the mindset that promotes true healing. Whatever we feed into our bodies is, in part, what they become. Remember the fashionable saying, "you are what you eat." A healthy mental diet is the keynote of Apple. This essence can help us to remain always calmly active and actively calm. While a diet of fresh fruits, vegetables, and whole grains is health-promoting to the body, so also a mental diet of courage, wisdom, and happiness is clarifying to the mind and the feelings of the heart.

"I took Apple for fear of a repeat experience," explained a chiropractor of forty years of age and working on clarity related to his physical constitution. "Three months ago, I suffered a mild stroke with resultant motor loss in my right hand. I experienced four strokes in five days from a narrowing of the carotid artery. This was unexplainable since I've had low cholesterol all my life and have been a strict vegetarian since I was eighteen."

The doctor admitted to a serious fear of illness and disability, saying that he would rather lose his life than the use of his hands. "I use my hands to heal and I love my work. Literally within half an hour of taking Apple, my mental clarity returned. I felt safe and whole and that I would get better. The healing was dramatic from that point on. I experienced a really strong sense of inner well-being." He also reported that he has regained ninety percent movement and usage of his right hand.

The positive Apple state reveals an understanding of the importance of clarity on all levels—a spiritual diet of meditation, proper breathing, and uplifting company and reading material; a certain brightness to our thought processes; and health-promoting exercise, diet, and living habits to restore us to perfect well-being.

People who are strong in the positive Apple qualities are often drawn to health-related work fields, including physically, psychologically, or spiritually. Their clarity of energy is invigorating to their clients and friends.

Apple is also indicated for recovery periods after surgery, illness, or accidents—or any time we are wanting to regain the subtle balance between the body, mind and spirit. "I muscle-tested (kinesiology) much stronger with Apple," one man wrote following a hip replacement surgery. "When I started taking it, I felt much better."

NEGATIVE INDICATIONS

Apple deals directly with the law of magnetism. When we embrace mental and physical health, we draw to ourselves more of the same. When we live with a lack of peace, we draw exactly that. When we catch that flu that's been going around—the one that took half the office staff by surprise—it may be the magnet of our own fear and resultant sense of susceptibility that opens the door and invites it in! If your attitude is, "Oh, I'm going to get sick, I just know it"—you're probably going to be right, just as you predicted.

The negative Apple state manifests as "the fear that magnetizes fear," especially if infused with enough energy. In fact, we could even define fear as a negative wish, phrased as innocently as, "Gee, I hope I don't get sick." Have you ever experienced a fear of:

- a problem recurring
- a communicable or terminal illness
- catching that "something going around"
- an imagined illness with no substantiation (hypochondria)
- diseases we read or hear about
- illnesses to which we are genetically predisposed

Add to this list any worry, doubt, or the absence of mental clarity, and we have the indications for taking Apple. Remember that the presence of any one of the above thought patterns is reason enough to administer this clarity-promoting essence.

THEME CHARACTERISTICS

The Apple theme, then, personifies mental health with an understanding of the subtle integration of body, mind, and soul. "Keeping the body fit for Self-realization" is understood by these themes. You may find them outside gardening as they work the soil with gloveless hands, both drawing the earth's nourishment and imbuing it into the seeds being planted. Apple themes embody healthy attitudes. Like Corn themes, they overflow with energy, though Apple's energy is directed more toward mental attitudes.

Apple themes have a certain gloss to their skin and a glow in their eyes. Their inner radiance vibrationally encourages others to live in a similar manner. Their example of healthy thoughts is very magnetic, and they make good team players in sports, in relationships, and on the job. If you feel under the weather, spend time with an Apple theme, a living example of calm activity.

FAMOUS THEME PERSONALITIES

Charles Atlas
George Beinhorn
Jack LaLaine
Sandow
Jane Fonda
Florence Griffith Joyner
Tom McMillen
J. I. Rodale
Bernard Jensen
Bernie Siegel

Any child who read comic books during the 1950's knows the name Charles Atlas. Apple theme magnetism literally radiates on a global level from his stunning, superstar physique! Responsible for the classic before-and-after ads of the skinny kid on the beach, Mr. Atlas offered a correspondence bodybuilding course employing techniques of dynamic tension. (An intriguing side note is that Yogananda admitted teaching a famous bodybuilder how to develop muscle and strength without lifting weights by directing will power through the use of kinesthetic "dynamic tension." Although their connection is at best implied, the timing and nature of the material are too uncanny to ignore. A similar program called the Energization Exercises is available in illustrated poster form from Ananda Village.)

Changing his given name from Angelo Siciliano to that of the mythological Greek Titan who held the heavens on his shoulders, Mr. Atlas helped transform the model of bodybuilding from the grosser, barrel-shaped strongman to the well-defined and proportioned aesthetic image of today. Mr. Atlas, an exemplary Apple theme, understood that the body is virtually manufactured by the mind. He demonstrated that the use of will power and energy create our physical temples and shape our mental altars.

CONFESSIONS OF AN APPLE THEME: WAYNE'S STORY

"I guess my general personality traits are that I can be extremely independent, totally content to operate on my own, and have lots of energy, especially for seclusive activities. I have a sort of superabundant energy most of the time.

"I'm so much into athletics now, and that gives me lots and lots of energy. When I'm running, I feel fine. I've noticed a difference from when I was younger. Now that I'm over fifty, there's a very great mental difference that affects my running and my feelings as I run. You know, many ultra-marathon runners are older—they're in their forties and fifties. There's probably a very psychological reason why that's true. The miles go by very differently when you're older and less attached to each mile. It's an interesting thing, more contemplative. The scenery just passes in a sort of pleasant fashion. You don't get all irritated because there is a hill or whatever. There's more of a flow.

"I am working on perfecting within myself the childlike qualities of joy and the heart—willingness to be enthusiastic about the next thing that needs to be done, and to do it happily and willingly. I want to overcome all the little hesitancies that stand in the way. My biggest worry right now is that I'll really get out of tune and lose whatever joy I've got or that I'll lose hope or my ability to love. And the biggest theme in my life is that of doubt, a kind of mental doubt. In the recent past, though, I think I've made some strides to get past that.

"I have a really indomitable kind of positive view of the future, that it holds all kinds of wonderful opportunities. I don't want to lose that, ever. No matter what kind of mistakes you make, I figure it's always possible to bob to the surface. I would not ever want to be depressed to the point that I lose that. . .that hope.

"Do I like apples? Oh, yeah! I mean, apple's my favorite fruit, my favorite food. My relationship to apples? I've eaten them consistently all year round, all of my life."

WRAPPING IT UP

Surely it is no coincidence that apples, of all fruits, occupy such a prominent place in folklore throughout time. In Greek and Roman mythology, the apple is a symbol of wealth, beauty, and the sun and moon. American folk medicine recommended using the apple to cure toothache, breast cancer, gonorrhea, as well as the emotional illness of melancholy.

The saying that "one bad apple spoils the whole bunch" could easily refer to the poisoning effect of one bad thought on our body and mind. Healthy attitudes, like a bushel of crisp, ripe apples, are the vibrational message of Apple. Keeping the mind, and likewise the body, "calmly active and actively calm" is of paramount importance to us all.

APPLE	*Contrasted With:*	*Companioned With:*
Blackberry	for negative thoughts of others	for a pure and healthy attitude toward oneself and others
Corn	for more general mental vitality	for a dynamic, unblocked flow of energy
Tomato	for overcoming non-health health-related fears	for confidence in one's abilities to overcome obstacles, especially mental blocks

Positive Expressions

Healthy in attitudes	Accepting
Positive-thinking	Whole
Fearless	Balanced
Strong	Well-beingness
Integrated in body/mind/spirit	Happy

Negative Conditions

Doubting	Prone to recurring negative
Given to unhealthy attitudes	emotions
Feeling impure	Indecisive
Feeling unclean	Fearful, specifically health-related
Tending toward hypochondria	Vulnerable
Worrying	

Essence Enhancers

Repeat the Apple affirmation several times a day, especially when feeling a lack of clarity.

Practice the Apple visualization whenever you feel the need.

Eat "an apple a day," and associate the crisp freshness of its taste and texture with the clarity of your thoughts.

Spend ten minutes a day in direct sunlight with a good sunscreen, either in the early morning or late afternoon. Consciously draw the sun's healing energy into your mind and body.

VISUALIZATION

For this visualization, you'll either need to be out in direct sunlight, or to imagine that you are.

Now, sit on a patch of grass. Place your palms face down beside you, directly on the greenery. Connect with the earth. Feel its magnetism of strength and solidity flowing into your palms, up your arms and radiating throughout your entire body. You and the earth are one. Its wholeness is yours.

Now turn your palms comfortably upward in such a way that they can receive the sunlight pouring into them. Be as receptive as possible, much like an empty vessel. Draw in the sunlight. Let its healing rays find a home in your hands. Through the posture of upturned palms, imagine that your entire consciousness is uplifted, broadened, and expanded. Feel your body, mind, and spirit drinking deeply of this direct source of life force. The flow of your thoughts has become as clear as the sunlight.

AFFIRMATION

With a crisp, clear attitude toward life I view my problems with ever fresh solution-consciousness.

CHAPTER TWENTY-FOUR

ORANGE: "THE SMILE MILLIONAIRE"

Citrus sinensis
("sweet common orange
from China")

"I was trying to wean my two-and-a-half-year-old son. He got really depressed and cranky. I gave him two drops of Orange for two days, and he was completely fine."

—*SJ, Norfolk, VA*

"My two-year-old son was teething—very sullen and whiny. Since he was eating nothing but oranges—orange slices, orange juice, orange popsicles—I started him on Orange essence. Wonderful results!"

—*LB, North San Juan, CA*

"I had a depressed childhood—dysfunctional, sexual abuse, the works. I am also overweight and dealing with Chronic Fatigue Syndrome. I like taking Orange. It helped me go through my therapy in a flash."

—*DDG, Long Beach, CA*

"I was depressed for a few days. I finally took Orange in the middle of the night. During my depression, my knee and hip went out, and I was limping around the house. Within minutes of taking Orange, my knee adjusted itself and hasn't bothered me since. Also, I felt my energy rising and felt like meditating—so I did. I kept taking the Orange for a few days—but the bulk of the problem was gone instantly."

—*MK, North San Juan, CA*

"But mortal bliss will never come sincere; Pleasure may lead,

but grief brings up the rear."   —Greek epigram

FLOWER/FRUIT/FOLKLORE

Originating in China and southeast Asia, the subtropical orange fruit dates back to at least 500 B.C. The small orange tree—a winged, leafy-stalked evergreen—grows to about twenty-five feet in height. Its tiny white flowers grow in clusters and exude a delicious scent. More than two hundred varieties of this "liquid sunshine" are grown in the US alone. Oranges, the famous immune boosters, are known as one of the best sources of water-soluble vitamin C. They aid the intestines, teeth, and gums.

Qualities: Enthusiasm, Hope

Message of Self-mastery: Energy; banishing melancholy; cultivating an inner smile; resolution of conflict; lightness; emotional integration; "light at the end of the tunnel"; renewed interest in life; for the power to endure difficulties.

Pattern of Disharmony: Mild to severe depression; hopelessness; despair; self-pity; for past or present abuse issues—physical, emotional, or sexual; apathy; the "might as well get used to it" attitude.

SPECTRUM PLACEMENT

Orange brings us to Quadrant III's final house. Also the last house of the Spectrum's masculine half, it resounds with the message of a zeal of great depth and strength, unlike the softer, lighter energy of Cherry. Clear-thinking Apple provides the psychologically balanced soil from which Orange germinates. Just as the fruit of the orange possesses a particular tartness, so do many of life's experiences. Determined to overcome the deepest possible human sorrows, Orange reaches to the very core of true happiness.

POSITIVE APPLICATIONS

Certain individuals are able to take trauma and crisis in stride; others buckle under and suffer greatly. Some children do better with teething than others. Some of the elderly, although understandably lonely, weather the passing of a spouse better than others. This leads us to the conclusion that it is not the experience itself, but the way we choose to react to it—similar to Cherry—that indicates the need for Orange. Culturally, we are faced with some shocking statistics on depression.

- Clinical depression affects twenty to thirty percent of adults at some time during their lives.
- The lifetime risk of suicide from major depressive disorders is fifteen percent, which is a higher mortality rate than that of many medical disorders.
- Depression and anxiety disorders are twice as common in women than in men. In women, the mid-thirties and forties represent the peak period of new-onset depression and anxiety.

I remember one particular afternoon of consultations following a morning Spirit-in-Nature workshop. Four people in a row came into the office and recounted their life stories of serious childhood abuse issues. One man was then suicidal; one woman had chosen a homosexual lifestyle that was proving problematic; another gentleman was undergoing long-term psychotherapy; one woman with a difficult childhood had become an elementary school teacher. All had suffered similar abusive situations and had adapted according to their own distinct personalities. Each individual, however, indicated the need for Orange.

Positive Orange is the loving parent by whom we may not have had the opportunity to be raised, who gently takes us by the hand and says, "This is a tough test, but you're going to be okay. We'll just see this through and come out the other side."

Orange is the essence of choice for those heavier-than-Cherry moods or chronic sadness. "I took Orange to dispel moods after a serious accident where I sustained a concussion," Patrick wrote. "I was told it would take time for the brain to heal, and to be patient. On Orange, I was able to get though the post-trauma weeks with little or no problem caused by down moods. I was also very steady with my emotions—in fact, steadier than I have been at other times when I wasn't going through a healing phase."

Negative Indications

Orange embodies the vibration of not giving up, or giving in, no matter how convincing the case in favor of despair. Orange is indicated for any experience that leaves us feeling as though we can't go on— the death of a loved one, divorce, miscarriage, thoughts of suicide, a disfiguring accident, or surgery or a chronic, lingering illness. Orange embodies hope and leads us through even the most long-term suffering to the light at the end of the tunnel.

One in the negative Orange state is far beyond the help of Cherry. The negative Cherry state may be likened to waking up on the wrong side of the bed; negative Orange is more like waking up on the wrong side of your life. Orange is helpful for long-standing problems—or long-term, counterproductive attitudes in dealing with those problems.

The negative Orange state, especially when prolonged, is that "end of one's rope" feeling. It may also indicate the need for other modalities of therapy in addition to taking Orange. (A word of caution: *flower essences do not replace proper medical attention.*) "I'd been depressed all day," Verna admitted. "I don't usually get depressed, but there it was. I was so depressed that I didn't even want to close up shop. I was going to binge on a box of cookies. Instead, I prayed for an answer and went right over to the Spirit-in-Nature Essences display. I picked up a bottle of Orange and felt better with the first dosage. I took it the next day too. The feeling of sadness disappeared."

The dictionary defines depression as a hollow or low place. Certainly for all of us, this describes those times in our lives when we have felt empty inside and hopeless. In the negative Orange state, it is easy to find justification for this absence of enthusiasm. Orange is like a "vibrational fork-lift" that scoops us out of the doldrums.

THEME CHARACTERISTICS

Orange wood is known for its flexibility, symbolic of the Orange theme's resilience in the face of monumental trials. Four or five ripe oranges will significantly bend a limb without snapping it—hence its popularity as a wood used in bow-making. Orange themes, likewise, may suffer greatly yet survive joyfully.

They are easily spotted by a certain heaviness or slowness to their movements. (Although this is a general rule, exceptions are not uncommon. Some Orange themes are very light-footed.) A history of difficulty throughout life, coupled with the stamina to overcome, creates their portfolio. Orange themes are survivors and, for this reason, make deeply inspirational company. You will feel their profound sense of inner bliss and hope gained through not one, but repeated, trials. In living so valiantly, they *become* the light at the end of the tunnel.

The delicate perfume of the orange blossom calls to mind the odor of sanctity, a scent said to exude from the bodies of saints. Orange themes are life's valiant saints. Purified in the fires of colossal tests, they emerge indomitably serene.

FAMOUS THEME PERSONALITIES

Ananda Moi Ma

St. Francis of Assisi

Betty Ford

Red Buttons

Rose Kennedy

Victor Frankl

Elizabeth Taylor

Charlie Chaplin

Mira Bai

"Joy-permeated Mother" is the name Yogananda bestowed upon Ananda Moi Ma, a Bengali saint. Although saints wear their theme essences thinly, their personalities purified of baser qualities, still we see sparse remnants of their themes. In his autobiography, Yogananda describes meeting the woman saint, her face "burnished with the ineffable joy that had given her the name of Blissful Mother." [10] An Orange theme of extraordinary magnitude, her mere presence so uplifted people that it effected many miraculous healings.

The lives of saints abound with many stories; one will have to suffice for us here. Born in 1896 in the heart of rural Bengal, Ma's sunny childhood temperament earned her the nicknames, *Hasi* ("smiles") and *Khusir Ma* ("the happy one"). Only on a few occasions did she ever cry, after the deaths of each of her three younger brothers, aged seven to several weeks. Witnessing the torrents of her mother's grief, she too broke into sobs. This caused her mother to cease crying and comfort the little girl who, by example, taught her mother that "grief brings up the rear" of all human experiences unless transmuted into true inner joy. In her later years, Ananda Moi said, "Whenever you have the chance, laugh as much as you can. By this all the rigid knots in your body will be loosened. But to laugh superficially is not enough: your whole being must be united in laughter, both outwardly and inwardly."[11] Yogananda wrote of the greatest heights of Orange, so beautifully attained by this Orange theme, in his famous poem entitled "Samadhi": "From joy I came, for joy I live, in sacred joy I melt."[12]

CONFESSIONS OF AN ORANGE THEME: JACK SHARES

"My childhood? Well, I was raised first by my grandmother and grandfather. My folks had split up and my mother left me in the care of my grandfolks while she was off working somewhere. When I was eight or ten, somewhere in there, my grandmother died, so my mother returned. I was raised by her the rest of the way. I lived mostly by myself. I was pretty much a loner, and learned to do things on my own. In school, it was not that I didn't enjoy the schoolwork, but I didn't enjoy being around other children that much. My childhood wasn't terribly unhappy, though.

"My emotions? I tend to suppress them. I'd say I'm a happy person, though. Why not? No, I wouldn't say I've had a hard life. I've had no more things to overcome than other people have—less than many—so I wouldn't say it was difficult. I've often seen myself struggling in situations where, looking back on it, I didn't need to struggle that hard. So there's often been a feeling in my life of struggle or pressure and effort. But I wouldn't call that being a hard life. It's just an expression of the energy one needs to get something out of life, to do something with it.

"Yes, I dealt with depression in the earlier part of my life. The first few years out of high school and college and through my twenties, I was often depressed until I started meditating and began to pull out of it. There were still a few periods of depression after that, but they gradually disappeared.

"Years ago when I lived in Arizona, I really enjoyed oranges. I bought them by the case and went on orange juice fasts. I would drink a ton of orange juice. I enjoy them a lot. I've been away from oranges lately. But usually about once or twice a year, I'll go get a bag of oranges. I'm not interested in the frozen juice and I'd rather have fresh juice than eat the orange."

WRAPPING IT UP

Studies conducted at Yale University Hospital have shown that there is a chemical in the oil of the orange that acts as an antidepressant. Similarly, the ultimate and timeless statement of Orange in flower essence form is that life is a dream. Loved ones will forever pass in and out of our lives, touching and transforming us in their own unique ways. A parade of events will endlessly shift before our gaze, like bits of glass in a kaleidoscope. Today's sorrow will be but a passing memory tomorrow, just as yesterday's greatest pleasure is now but a pleasant souvenir of the moment.

Yes, we may have suffered serious abuse at the hands of the ignorant or the unwise. But this, too, can pass. Our lesson is to learn kindness from the unkindness of others, and to move forward with hope. Orange's song, then, is the joy of living, loving, and letting go. With enthusiasm, we can transmute resignation and bitterness into acceptance. The poverty of a sense of loss becomes the vast richness of experience that brings us more perfectly into alignment with our own highest potential.

ORANGE	Contrasted With:	Companioned With:
Avocado	for thoughts and emotions that cloud our mental outlook	for remembering that joy is the core of our life
Cherry	for passing moods	for an energetic understanding that joy on all levels is our true nature
Coconut	perseverance through a wide range of tests not necessarily involving depression	stamina with tests that are especially heavy or emotionally trying
Pear	for emotional balance	for the ability to survive trying times no matter how severe; for major catastrophic events
Spinach	to aid the inner child who suffered an unhappy childhood	to vibrationally remove the residual effects of a dysfunctional childhood

POSITIVE EXPRESSIONS

Joyful	Hopeful
Transcendent	Energetic
Enthusiastic	Expressing the power to endure
Persevering	Vital
Resilient	Renewing interest in life
Blissful	Light
Serene	Smiling from within

NEGATIVE CONDITIONS

Sad	Melancholic
Heavy	Lacking in energy
Apathetic	Feeling burdened
Resigned	Despairing
Disinterested	Hopeless
Negative	Irresolute

ESSENCE ENHANCERS

Seek counseling or other forms of constructive help.

Connect with a support group to band with others going through similar difficulties.

Join an organization where you can give help and support to those who are going through the same or similar kinds of tests that you have overcome.

Practice viewing your life—especially the particularly difficult parts—as a passing dream. Do so without reacting emotionally, as if it's someone else's life you are observing.

Find happiness in the little things in your life, gradually expanding to bigger ones; reading a favorite book, planting a flower garden or jogging with your dog.

VISUALIZATION

For this exercise, you will need to stand in front of a mirror.

Look into the reflection of your eyes. What do you see there? Are they laughing, sad, contented, or disgruntled? Now look at the shape of your face—its contours, its features, the texture and color of your skin, and the way you hold your head and shoulders. What does your posture tell you about yourself? Would you say your are self-confident? One-pointed? Contented?

Having assessed your body language and facial expression, place the tip of each index finger at the corners of your mouth, all the while studying the face staring back at you. Push the corners of your mouth upward, forming a smile of sorts, or at least the beginning of one. Now place your hands at your sides, maintaining the expression. Allow the smile to glide over the contours of your face like a cloud leaving a sun-lit trail in its wake on a hillside. In the physical process of smiling, let your face be bathed in the exhilaration of this smile.

Watch your reflection as the smile reaches your eyes. Observe the change in your energy, your posture, and finally your heart. Now, repeat the following affirmation.

AFFIRMATION

My thoughts dance on air with cosmic energy. Singing joyfully, they "soar" above every dark valley of sorrow!

CHAPTER TWENTY-FIVE

BLACKBERRY:
"THE ALL-PURPOSE
PURIFIER"

Rubus alleghenienses
("wild berries from
the Alleghenies")

"I am production and shipping manager in a small gift store. I have to admit I am extremely emotional and tend to go through severe PMS depression, weepiness, and fear. I'm also very hard on myself that I call the 'woe-is-me' syndrome. After three days on Blackberry, I experienced a new phenomena—a sense of humor! I've lightened up considerably—things aren't as bad as I thought."—*MM, Springdale, AR*

"Blackberry put me more in the moment and got me out of a state of denial. I felt this last week that I've gotten sane. Where *have* I been?"
— *CC, Plano, TX*

"On Blackberry, I experienced clearer thinking, sharper senses, faster speech—and a quick wit." —*RM, Dallas, TX*

"Blackberry was a blessed relief. I never felt so much power from an essence. I was so flat down before taking it!" —*AH, Albuquerque, NM*

"You know, if I don't take Blackberry in the afternoon, I sort of get rattled. But if I do, I don't get short-tempered with my four-year-old."
—*VY, Nevada City, CA*

"Even from the body's purity, the mind receives a secret, sympathetic aid."   —James Thomson

FLOWER/FRUIT/FOLKLORE

Blackberries, classified into two hundred species, are native to North America and Europe, and are now cultivated in every part of the United States. These hardy climbing plants produce fruit in large clusters at the ends of the older shoots. They survive two to three years. The delicate flowers of this prickly-stemmed bramble fruit are small and a pale lavender-pink in color. Blackberries are high in iron, calcium, and phosphorus and are excellent blood builders and bowel regulators. Blackberry leaf tea purifies the blood, heart, and skin.

Quality: Purity of Thought

Message of Self-mastery: Kindness; mental clarity; optimism; seeing goodness within oneself and others; inspirational; incisive and direct, yet gentle in speech; offended by mistreatment of living things; environmental awareness; for purification; for "sloughing off the old."
Pattern of Disharmony: Negativity; pessimism; sarcasm; cynicism; focus on dark and unkind thoughts with resultant downward flow of energy; fault-finding nature; bluntness; tactlessness.

SPECTRUM PLACEMENT

Blackberry heralds entry into the fourth and final Quadrant, that of winter and senior years. In this house we also return to the feminine half of the Spectrum. Thus these last five essences all possess a certain softness, gentleness, and kindness, with the transitional Blackberry revealing the masculine quality of discrimination. Although innocent in a childlike way, Blackberry bespeaks the depth and maturity of the fourth Quadrant. This Quadrant marks the beginning of a retreat into the self to store lessons learned, much like Nature withdrawing into the earth as winter approaches.

Blackberry thematically encapsulates the energy of its predecessor, Orange. Internalizing Orange's deep happiness and purified in its fires of great trials, Blackberry captures the quality of purity through the presence of light and goodness. It claims a clarity based on honest self-assessment and self-understanding. In addition, it promotes the wisdom of maturity rather than the innocence of inexperience and thus the ability to emerge from life's trials with a purity and clarity of logic and feeling alike.

POSITIVE APPLICATIONS

The positive Blackberry state offers us the vibrational imprint of clarity, focus, and the ability to see things as they really are—the antithesis of darkness, mental cloudiness, and denial, respectively. Blackberry's is an innocence, not born of ignorance, but rather of its opposite—knowledge through experience. A mind free from judgment, prejudice, and negativity epitomizes Blackberry.

When we judge or blame ourselves, or have a sense of uncleanliness for things that we have said or done in the past and can no longer change, Blackberry is indicated. This essence helps us to see events as dreams that have ended, allowing us to move forward with a clean slate, as it were.

"When I use Blackberry with its affirmation, it helps me clear out emotions such as resentment," Mario writes. "It has always worked in this regard."

The positive Blackberry state is exemplified by those who are environmentally aware. You will never catch these people littering! They tend to be politically informed, well-read, well-educated, and conscientious in their decisions. You will find them in animal rights groups; performing community service; or sorting and recycling their newspapers, glass bottles, and plastic containers. In addition to cleaning up the environment, they like to purify themselves as well, through fasting and cleansing diet regimens.

The highest octave of Blackberry can be seen as a "deep and meaningful relationship" with truth. Self-honesty is a must; honesty from others is assumed. Blackberry is the cut-to the-chase essence—direct, yet kindly; tactful, but to the point.

NEGATIVE INDICATIONS

The negative Blackberry state is seen in those whose emotional natures have not yet matured, and who may, even inadvertently, let slip unkind words. Those who behave with cynicism, sarcasm or negativity—in short, the carping spirit—are expressing the need for Blackberry Essence.

Individuals in the negative Blackberry state have nothing nice to say about anyone or anything. They are prone to gossip and tend to tell offensive, racist, or prejudicial jokes at the expense of others, especially those forced to listen to them. Often without realizing it, they create a foul, repellent energy around themselves, making them difficult company for very long.

"My husband of twenty-one years has a 'sour grapes' attitude," Lisbeth shared, somewhat reluctantly. "When we moved to the Midwest, nothing in our new home pleased him. The curtains were stale-looking, the neighbors were too noisy, and the walls too thin, according to him. I took Blackberry because his negativity seemed so contagious. Within a few days, I began to see goodness all around me. I learned to deflect his comments with my optimism. My appreciation of life increased a hundredfold."

A milder version of the negative Blackberry state is found in the individual who, quite without realizing it, is simply unpleasant to be around. There may be hints of a Cherry mood, or the strong, negative emotions of Lettuce, but the Blackberry state leaves one feeling somehow unclean, as though missing the boat of life's loveliness.

Blackberry is also the essence for frustration, a state we all experience from time to time. When our thoughts are confused or conflicted, or when our energy isn't flowing, Blackberry helps to clean the mud from our mental window.

THEME CHARACTERISTICS

Blackberry themes will oftentimes have very sharp and striking facial features. Their eyes may be piercing and they will look straight into yours when speaking to you. They are direct in speech and do not "beat around the bush." You may find them pausing between sentences, searching for just the right words to express their thoughts, or they may correct themselves from time to time, similar to Fig themes, for truth is of paramount importance to them.

Blackberry themes keep track of their thoughts. Vigilant and always conscious, they are aware of how these thoughts affect themselves and those around them. Because they magnetically invite self-scrutiny and honesty, they make excellent counselors or progress rapidly in their own therapies. You will find them to be sincere and lasting friends. Are you feeling confused? Unclear? Spend time with Blackberry themes. In the sunlight of their refreshing purity, you will find fresh insights sprouting in your own mental garden.

FAMOUS THEME PERSONALITIES

Paracelsus
Barbara Walters
Martin Luther King, Jr.
Counselor Diana Troi
Louis Pasteur
Francis Bacon
Socrates
Lucy from "Peanuts" Cartoon
George Washington

Most telling of all Paracelsus' Blackberry theme traits is that the word, "bombast," originates from his given name, Philippus Theophrastus Bombastus von Hohenheim. Born near Zurich, Switzerland, this Renaissance physician (mentioned in Chapter Four) played an influential role in turning medical treatment toward a more scientific approach. He may have been the first to apply the concept of home-opathy in declaring that "what makes a man ill also cures him." His discoveries illustrates the Blackberry theme's commitment to truth, no matter what the response of his contemporaries.

Paracelsus was actually extremely unpopular with academics and physicians alike—to such a degree that he never stayed in one place very long! His incisive way with words made him many enemies and yet, as a brilliant diagnostician, he was greatly revered by his patients for his success and his kindness. Through his Blackberry-like desire to bring clarity and optimum results to the healing field, Paracelsus is credited with initiating many ground-breaking therapies. He was the first to use chemotherapy; to pioneer the use of mercury as a curative for syphilis; and to claim that miners' chest ailments were caused by inhalation of toxins rather than evil spirits. This opinionated and out-spoken spokesman of medical science exemplifies a truly illuminating Blackberry theme.

CONFESSIONS OF A BLACKBERRY THEME: BRETT'S TALE

"It was a good childhood, but it was also very guarded and pro-tected. There was some emotional abuse. My parents did the best they could. I've done a lot of self-work. Of course, there are still issues that I'm working on. But as I'm being more clear, more aware of what the issues are, I can catch myself and see them when they come up, and then I have a choice of what to do from there.

"I'm a yoga instructor by profession. I have a fairly active mind. It tends to be a bit of a busybody. I seem to pay too much attention to details. I'm trying to be more and more open to my emotions. I grew up in a culture where it's not okay to have emotions, especially if they're not positive. I really had to look at this when I first started taking responsibility for myself.

"I'm not an extrovert or a very social person. Social chitchatting is very hard for me to do. I'm not comfortable in those situations where it feels very forced just to say something. I like to have some kind of meaningful interaction with good friends, or even with people I don't know very well. I feel it's a waste of time otherwise. That's my nature.

"I really admire people who are open and that I know where they are at all times, who are truthful with themselves and others. So you always know what's going on. That's really important to me.

"I think I picked a harder lifetime, maybe because by doing so I have a chance to grow more. If things came too easily for me, maybe I wouldn't put the energy into it that I've had to do this way. I know that in my nature, the things I have to watch out for are being judgmental, critical, analytical. And I always work consciously on not going in a negative direction. For most of my life, I was too afraid to ask people for truth and clarification, so people thought I was confrontational. I'm better at it now.

"I like blackberries. I haven't really been around them much since I've been in this country. But I used to, and still do, really like berries— more than other fruits."

WRAPPING IT UP

The quality of purity, Yogananda said, is inherent in all berries except raspberry and strawberry—these two excel in other elevating traits. I selected blackberries from which to make the Spirit-in-Nature Essence for this quality. Blackberry's energy is clean, straight forward, trustworthy, and above all, pure. Bordering the horizon of the Spectrum's masculine and feminine halves, it integrates clear reason with pure feeling.

"Cleanliness is next to Godliness," the saying goes. The desire for a clean environment and a pure, orderly mind are typical Blackberry traits. Remember that this remedy has a tendency to make things look worse, or larger, than they really are—anger in particular. The truth is, Blackberry only makes us more aware of our negative traits. Being ready and willing to look at our "stuff" is actually a very positive sign and is the first step in being able to clear it from our consciousness. You may find Blackberry's silent slogan on your car's side view mirror: "Objects are closer than they appear."

BLACKBERRY	*Contrasted With:*	*Companioned With:*
Apple	for worried and fearful thoughts	for a pure and healthy attitude toward oneself and others
Cherry	for moods rather than negative thoughts	for pure happiness
Lettuce	for strong negative emotions such as anger and resentment	for creative, focused mental clarity

POSITIVE APPLICATIONS
Pure
Innocent
Having a sense of humor
Clear
Sincere
Direct
Truthful
Ability to focus
Sharp-thinking
Self-honest
Articulate
Moral in character
Honorable
Discriminating
Common-sensical
Mature
Frugal
Kind
Self-studying
Insightful
Introspective
Clean
Straightforward

NEGATIVE CONDITIONS
Cynical
Sarcastic
Negative
Pessimistic
Mean
Cruel
Insulting to self or others
Unkind with humor
Gossipy
Denial-prone
Judgmental
Closed-minded
Tactless
Prone to clouded thinking
Fault-finding
Blunt
Feeling unclean
Self-blaming
Evasive
Confrontational
Deceptive
Dishonest
Frustrated
Outrageous
Prone to dark thoughts

ESSENCE ENHANCERS

At the end of the day, read the Blackberry list of *Positive Expressions/Negative Conditions*. Place a check mark next to the qualities you experienced. Assess accordingly whether you need to upgrade your "mental wardrobe."

Read self-help books about subjects you are trying to excel in.

At bedtime, fill your mind with pleasant, uplifting thoughts to penetrate the subconscious mind.

Make it a point to focus on the inherent goodness in the people around you.

VISUALIZATION

Autumn has barged in so quickly, pushing summer in her pastel gossamer into a muted corner. Mother Nature tucks in all the green lace of warmer seasons, replacing it with crisp, crackly colors—colors that bite, colors that sing from a distance now.

The midday sun feels warm on the nape of your neck, and the country trail sprawling before you hasn't known human footprints for many cycles of seasons. The vine-laden blackberry bushes extend their berry-filled branches to you, like gnarled hands with thorns for long, sharp fingernails. The berries seem to be smiling at you, all dark-hued and juicy. Their thorny protection makes the picking process one of caution and not to be undertaken absentmindedly.

The more berries you pick and tuck into your shirttails, the more wine-stained are your hands. The ripe ones fall almost eagerly into your palms, and just as readily into your mouth. Puckeringly tart and seedy, the juice purifies both your blood and your thoughts.

The more berries you eat, the more you reflect on the psychological nature of this wild fruit. The seeds are like seed thoughts—fresh ideas, pure insights, and clear observations. The purifying pulp of the fruit both cleanses and builds you at the same time. And the thorns are incisive admonitions to live cleanly in body and mind.

Nourished and cleansed by this welcome snack, you continue on your walk.

AFFIRMATION

Pure thoughts, like rays of sunlight, penetrate the dust-covered windows of my mind. They fill me with good will toward all.

CHAPTER TWENTY-SIX

DATE:
"THE CONSCIOUS COOKIE JAR"

Phoenix dactylifera ("fingerlike date palm")

"1 feel I've suffered many disappointments since my mother died, especially in my friendships. On Date, I found that I was able to wish people well. It's as if a new person were emerging from inside of me. It's a wonderful feeling!"
—*AL, Albuquerque, NM*

"On Date Essence, I felt an invisible inner sweetness extending from myself to others. I got tears in my eyes from taking it. It melted my critical wall."
—*KC, Cedarburg, WI*

"Date helped my eight-year-old son find an inner sweetness that he thought could only come from eating sugar. Rarely do I let him eat white sugar, and rarely does he ask for it. But this morning, he was demanding it. We had just moved from the city to the country, and he was quite homesick for his friends. I gave him the Date to help his emotional sweet tooth, and the craving quit within hours."
—*MS, Mesquite, TX*

"I took Date for a sugar craving which then lightened up a bit. But what was interesting was that my taking Date made three of my friends more aware of the need for sweetness in their own lives."
—*JR, Mountain View, CA*

"I put Date in my husband's tea, and he just really softened. He even joined a self-help group!"
—*CR, Novato, CA*

"Sweet speaking oft a currish heart reclaims." —Sir Philip Sidney

Flower/Fruit/Folklore

The subtropical date palm was first cultivated in Mesopotamia and the Nile Valley of Egypt over five thousand years ago. For centuries, Arabian caravans relied upon dried dates as their principal food source on long journeys across the desert. Reaching a height of about eighty feet, a healthy tree will yield one hundred fifty pounds of dates per year. The bright white male and female flowers being borne on separate plants, only one male tree is necessary to pollinate fifty to one hundred female trees. Dates are a good source of copper, calcium, phosphorus, iron—and calories. They contain sixty to seventy percent sugar and thus are a readily available source of energy. Dates are considered an excellent digestive aid and laxative, as well as a folk remedy for some forms of cancer.

Quality: Tender Sweetness
Message of Self-mastery: Attunement to others' feelings; discrimination; receptivity; open-mindedness; easy to talk to; welcoming; a magnetic nature; for dealing kindly with the public; self-nurturance.
Pattern of Disharmony: Judgmental and critical of others; intolerance; unaccepting nature; for an easily irritated nature; unpleasant to be around; inhospitality.

Spectrum Placement

Having integrated Blackberry's ability to see goodness in everything and everyone, we become sweet. Hence, the evolution to Quadrant IV's second house, Date. Blackberry's clarity contributes to Date's ability to observe without judgment. Date's sweetness places it in the feminine half of the Spectrum; its maturity, in the Quadrant of a wintering, reflective agelessness.

POSITIVE APPLICATIONS

The positive side of Date expresses a warmth and amiability that draws people to us. Unconditional acceptance is a magnetic attitude with the power to illicit kindness from friends and strangers alike. The following is one of my all-time favorite Date stories.

"It wasn't until a friend recommended Date that I started to look at how judgmental and critical I am," wrote Peter. "I'm constantly finding fault with my girlfriend—it's a wonder she's still with me! Anyway, I took Date one night and felt different, though I can't say what it was. The next morning, I went out for my morning bike ride, and very strange things happened. Everybody—I mean *everybody*—was waving to me. Two strangers even stopped me just to chat! I continued on the Date, and for the next three weeks, friends I hadn't seen in years started calling, wanting to get together. I don't mean one or two—I mean about half a dozen."

The positive Date state is also one of tenderness. Often without knowing it, others feel embraced by our non-judgmental, unconditional love. "I guess the Date must be working," said Christina. "I started taking it this morning and, this afternoon, my husband kept smiling at me and telling me how *sweet* I looked. I may stay on this one a long time!"

This is one of my all-time favorite reports: "I use Date every weekend to be nice to my boyfriend. We've been dating—no pun intended—for three months now and, although I love him dearly, he bores me to death. He's just set in his ways and doesn't want to change. I get irritable and testy, and then I start screaming at him. He still bores me, but on Date, I just put up with him."

Date and Peach share an interesting vibrational similarity. Both residents of the feminine half of the Spectrum, Peach symbolizes the young mother, whereas Date represents the indulgent grandmother, wont to spoil us at times with her sweet love. Date, then, helps us to understand that we are all a part of this human circus. Audience or actor, clown or acrobat—it's all the same. Without judgment, we become sweet. Without narrowness of vision, we can develop the quality of tenderness.

NEGATIVE INDICATIONS

The negative Date condition is anything but sweet. Here we see the miserly Scrooge who withholds his finer qualities from others and is irritable and irascible as well. In the negative state of Date, one becomes critical instead of discerning, judgmental rather than discriminating. He who succumbs to this state of mind finds himself without friends—lonely and, frankly, unlikable. In the negative Date condition, much like Blackberry, one unconsciously and successfully pushes others away.

Negative Date possesses a narrowness of attitude—egocentricity, or viewing everything in relation to oneself. Granted, sometimes people use themselves as a point of reference, but the concept infers a negative connotation when we choose to see the world as centered around ourselves, or when we expect others to be exactly like us.

From this vantage point, we are wont to compare. Others are, by nature, different from us. Before long, we are not only comparing but tagging value judgments onto those comparisons as well. "She's taller than me—how can I go out with her?" "He dresses funny—those styles were outdated years ago!" Now we find not only judgment but separation from others as a result of such narrow and unloving attitudes. These character pitfalls indicate the need for Date Essence.

THEME CHARACTERISTICS

Lest the Date theme become stereotyped as the jolly fat man or the cheek-pinching grandmother, this essence is far more subtle and thus easily mistaken for other themes. Date's is a sweetness quite unlike what Ring Lardner so humorously described in the man who "gave her a look that you could've poured on a waffle." Date themes are anything but syrupy; their compassion, wisdom, and empathy run deep.

The faces of these themes express a paradoxical softness and strength. You will see Blackberry's residual no-nonsense attitude coupled with Date's kindliness. Date theme voices are either soft and sweet like the fruit pulp or firm and strong like the pit. And as Spinach reveals the adult within the child, Date hints at the child within the elder. Date themes' movements and gait are both slow and quick at the same time. They readily magnetize sweetness and acceptance from those around them. Once experiencing the deep love flowing through them, we are encouraged to act likewise—sensitive to others, welcoming, and without judgment. These dear and loving individuals see the child within us all.

FAMOUS THEME PERSONALITIES

Santa and Mrs. Claus
Joan Plowright
Cinderella's fairy godmother
Good Witch in "The Wizard of Oz"
Snoopy
Charlie Brown
Ellen Burstyn
Mr. Rogers
Mr. Greenjeans
Harrison Ford
Sherry Lewis

Not to contradict the previous section, but the perfect embodiment of a Date theme is Santa Claus. Far beyond the simple nurturing of Peach, we find this timeless character digging into his bottomless sack of gifts—the greatest being the qualities of sweetness and tenderness. Santa sees the goodness in all children, without judging their naughtiness or niceness. To him, strangers and even enemies are family and friends. Santa, too, might reside in Quadrant IV of wintertime and ripening years—a place reminiscent of the North Pole. Santa exemplifies the physical Date theme characteristics of a sweet and kindly face, especially around the eyes. He radiates Date's approachableness and its loving nature.

Confessions of a Date Theme: Marilyn Speaks

"I would like to perfect acceptance within myself. I have a sense in this lifetime, because it has kept coming to me, that it is something that has been given to me to work on—especially given the great difficulty I have with acceptance. With acceptance comes understanding. I'm excited to say that I can look and see how much progress I've made. But at the same time I know that there's much more work that I need to do on myself. "I would say, yes, I tend toward judgmentalism. I have invited my friends and my partners to always call me on it because it's something that I want not to have present in my life. I was brought up in a very judgmental culture, first in Scotland. Scottish people tend to keep to themselves and think that they are, by far, superior to the English. Then I went to Africa where the whites think that they're superior to the blacks. And then I was with the Afrikaners who think that they are superior to the English!

"It's interesting that you should ask if I relate to the qualities of sweetness and tenderness because, when I came into this house, it was totally emptied out of everything that was here before—except for one place on the wall. There was a decorative card, and I felt like it was a message to me because it said 'tenderness.' And I thought, 'Where am I in regard to tenderness?' I realize that I'm very tender with children. My heart melts, even if they're acting out, cussing and swearing, and threatening. For years I ran a foster home for abused and abandoned children. I feel a deep tenderness and compassion for them. I know that they are not their behavior, that they are merely trying to tell me something about their deep pain.

"I also saw the same tenderness with my child and saw that I didn't have it with my partner or with myself. I tend to be very responsible. And sometimes when we're very responsible, we don't take the time to allow ourselves the tenderness. So I started seeing that as something I wanted to work on: to really be tender with my partner and also with myself.

"I see sweetness in babies and in animals. I hesitate to talk about sweetness because I do see people having an outward sweetness. One thing that I know about myself, and that people point out to me, is that I'm very solid. It's a very solid being that I feel inside myself.

"I love date fruits! When I spent time in the Arab countries, I traveled with the Bedouins and we ate dates. I loved that we got to the freshest source of them. We used to have them in Africa but they were imported and not the same at all."

WRAPPING IT UP

All five essences in Quadrant IV, though blanketed in snowy robes of winter's energy, carry a message of great strength—of gentleness, softness, and deep contentment. Pulpy on the outside, the date fruit's stone-like pit is symbolic of Date's core of unmistakable solidity. And the positive Date's refusal to be irritated by others reveals an acceptance of his own shortcomings as well as those of others.

A wise man once said that the craving for sweets is actually a desire for more sweetness in our lives. Sweetness can be synonymous with gratification. It is a pleasing taste; hence the popularity of candy, especially chocolate. Studies have confirmed a chemical in chocolate called phenylethylamine (PEA) that is also produced by the brains of people who are in love. How often we use sweets to create that sense of being in love, to fill that occasional void in our lives! In truth, what we are really seeking is a much deeper fulfillment. Date essence reminds us that we need not dip into the cookie jar for what we feel is lacking. The date fruit possesses a rich sweetness of its own—so rich that only a few are needed to satisfy our craving for sweets, even as only a few of Date's loving qualities make *us* sweet.

Through the vibration of non-judgment, Date allows us to make peace with ourselves and those around us—loved ones with whom we live day after day and those who seem to deliberately walk into our lives just to test us. Date awakens this truth that we already know: the sweetness we seek through rich desserts already lies within our own nature in abundance.

DATE	Contrasted With:	Companioned With:
Fig	critical of self, not others; a driving taskmaster	for balance through accepting oneself and others acknowledging imperfections with tolerance
Peach	for compassion	for sensitivity to others; for sweetening relationships

POSITIVE EXPRESSIONS

Sweet
Tender
Accepting
Sensitive
Discriminating *
Receptive
Open-minded
Contented
Welcoming

Magnetic
Discerning *
Drawing abundance
Compassionate
Wise *
Solid
Strong
Self-nurturing
Responsible

NEGATIVE CONDITIONS

Judgmental
Lonely
Irritable
Irascible
Craving sweets
Critical
Intolerant

Unaccepting
Unpleasant companion
Inhospitable
Sour
Discontented
Narrow
Annoyed

ESSENCE ENHANCERS

Develop the quality of hospitality—through having friends over for tea or dinner; by taking an official role as a greeter at your church, community center, or formal social event; or by participating in family get-togethers or reunions.

Observe how you relate to discourteous drivers while out in traffic. Improve on this if necessary, especially when they irritate you.

Do kindly things for friends and family, by anticipating their needs ahead of time—mending for a single friend or relative; bringing a cooked meal to someone who is ill; or delivering flowers to celebrate a birthday or house-warming.

VISUALIZATION

It's cold outside, colder than usual. You bundle up with hat, scarf, and mittens, without even being reminded by anyone—except the burst of snowflakes that blows in the door as you step out. Everything looks big, bigger than you remember. But that is because you have become very little. You find yourself in the prime of childhood.

The trees look taller, the snowdrifts along the sidewalk, higher. With a child's imagination, you know it's only a stone's throw to the North Pole. At every third or fourth step, you punch your boot into a pile of feathery snow, just to see how it feels.

There's the cabin now, built of stone as white as snow. The chimney lazily exhales a careless trail of smoke into the twilight sky. You knock on the door and are greeted by the legend himself. Although your eyes parallel the great round belt of the red-costumed man, already you feel welcomed and silently invited in. The scent of hot apple cider spiced with cinnamon sticks further entices you. Is it your imagination or is the room filled with the sound of laughter and sleigh bells?

Your child-eyes drink in the sweetness of a red-felt belly and a cascade of white beard and white hair escaping the red hat. But most of all you are caught up in the loving, laughing eyes of this living wonder whom youngsters have waited for and squealed for since the very first children sat on his lap and spilled out their wishes.

You know you can ask anything of old Saint Nick—toys, treasures, candy, or gold. In fact, just knowing that you *can* have whatever you ask for makes the asking a very serious matter indeed. What do you want? Toys, treasures, candy, or gold?

"Yes, Santa," you hear yourself saying. "I want all of these things in the form of sweetness that I may give them freely to others, young and old alike." He answers you, not with words, but with a very big, crinkly smile. And in that treasured smile is all the sweetness your heart has ever desired.

AFFIRMATION

I send waves of sweetness to everyone I meet.

CHAPTER TWENTY-SEVEN

STRAWBERRY:
"THE NOBLE ONE"

Fragaria chiloensis
("sweet-scented strawberry
of Chile")

"Strawberry not only helped me to support myself better but to understand my husband as well. On this essence I was able to know more of what his work means to him, his love for it—I couldn't before. It also allowed me to tell him that I wanted to move, that we are living in a place that doesn't work for me." — *UK, Plano, TX*

"I wanted to try your essences for my store. I found myself needing to get more grounded. I am very sensitive psychically and am too much out of my body. The Strawberry really got things moving and stabilized me. Results were very noticeable." —*JL, Guerneville, CA*

"I noticed a much more even energy on Strawberry—didn't get as bothered by things, like the children saying, 'I hate school and I'll never go again!'" —*AB, Nevada City, CA*

"I felt better, more centered, more confident. I teel like a different person! Strawberry gave me a different way of looking at myself. Something has changed—including my handwriting! It feels like a light came on that had been turned off for a long time."

—*VK, Nevada City, CA*

"I felt a difference in the first few days on Strawberry in that my attitude toward myself changed. The mental tapes I had been running were replaced by new, more uplifting ones. I could feel that at a *deep* subtle level, I was different. There were no other external changes to which I could attribute these results. Inwardly I had been trying for a long time without success." *JC, Sacramento, CA*

"But if a man happens to find himself. . .he has a mansion
which he can inhabit with dignity all the days of his life."

—James Michener

FLOWER/FRUIT/FOLKLORE

Strawberry belongs to the genus *Fragaria*, from the Latin word for fragrant, owing to the fruit's sweet smell. It is a member of the rose family. The strawberry originated in North and South America and early varieties date back to the 1500's. In 1643, Roger Williams said, "God could have made, but God never did make, a better berry." The strawberry, however, having no seeds within its fleshy pulp, is not classified as a true berry. A perennial herb with clusters of small leaves and white flowers, the strawberry plant grows low to the ground. Its runners will take root and grow new plants. The fruit is a good source of vitamin C, potassium, and fruit sugar. Fresh strawberries will remove tooth stains, soothe sunburn, and lighten freckles. High in dietary fiber, they are beneficial to the intestinal tract and are considered to be a "food of youth."

Quality: Dignity

Message of Self-mastery: Strong, quiet sense of self and self-worth; for grounding; reliability; for leaving a dysfunctional childhood in the past; poise; gracefulness; being fully present and comfortable in, and about, one's body.

Pattern of Disharmony: Guilt-ridden; low sense of self-worth; self-blaming; feeling unworthy, undeserving; irresponsible; being ungrounded; unsure of self; history of emotionally abusive parents; for psychic over-sensitivity; compares self to others, as in "why couldn't I be more like him."

SPECTRUM PLACEMENT

Located in the very mid-section of Quadrant IV, this essence embodies a feminine maturity, fullness, comfort, and poise. Date's sweetness has rendered us good-natured; now Strawberry makes us gracious and ennobled. This essence knows itself, but in a much more soft, quiet way than the conspicuous Pineapple. Strawberry, enriched by Quadrant IV's growing wisdom, loves the beauty of life, seeks it out, and finds it readily.

POSITIVE APPLICATIONS

Strawberry is especially helpful during times of transition, for these are the times when we are more likely to doubt ourselves. We may merely need to adjust to specific changes within our bodies or our environments: puberty, mid-life crisis, or menopause. Strawberry is also helpful during the dissolution of relationships; for the person who is left; and for the child dealing with a divorce. It helps us to remain present in the moment and deal with the issues at hand and, ultimately, to realize that all of our needs are met from within ourselves, thereby banishing a sense of lack.

Some years ago, a well known astrologer came for a consultation. The woman with whom he was deeply in love seemed unable to make a commitment to him. This situation was beginning to cause him much suffering. After one week on Strawberry, he decided that it was time to clarify the relationship and take a stand. He presented her with a choice; commit, or he was leaving. The stars were in his favor. She was impressed by his decisiveness. They have been married—happily, I'm told—for some time now.

There is much talk these days of self-esteem, a term defined as either belief in oneself or conceit. Strawberry's message—an important and oft-needed one in individual essence programs—is not so much to esteem ourselves as to walk, breathe, and speak from the state of our true source of loving dignity, which is divinity. Isn't this much better than merely esteeming ourselves?

NEGATIVE INDICATIONS

Strawberry embodies the issues that we all have to address at some time in our lives. Perhaps we suffer moments or possibly decades of self-doubt and unworthiness. Anything less than an ideal child-hood—that probably includes most of the human race—can foster problems with self-worth. Any time we fail at a task is a potential time of self-questioning. "I'm just not good enough"; "I can't do anything right"—these are thought patterns indicating the need for Strawberry. It is also the essence for self-blame, feelings of inadequacy, and guilt over many issues, including sexuality.

Strawberry-like self-worth issues are imprinted by parents on their children. Children, in turn reaching adulthood, recreate these patterns, possibly perpetuating generations of unhealthy family patterning. But with energy, insight, and grace, the dysfunctional spell may be broken. Strawberry is an excellent supportive remedy for freeing us from these deeply ingrained, hurtful patterns.

This essence vibrationally encourages the expression of grounding, centering and feeling integrated in our body, during adolescence in particular. It is helpful for children and adults who tend to be spacey, dreamy, or irresponsible. Because of its grounding effect, it strengthens those who are psychically oversensitive and need to be less affected by the energies of others.

THEME CHARACTERISTICS

Many years ago, I encountered a small girl, ten years at most, who beautifully personified the Strawberry theme. During my travels in India, I had the good fortune to spend several days aboard a houseboat on Kashmir's Dal Lake. This young girl, a saleswoman of sorts, spent her days paddling alongside the tourist *shikaras* (small, festive boats), selling freshly picked lotus blossoms. As she tossed flower clusters into our boat, I asked, "How much?" "Whatever you like," she replied in English, so unlike the other "hawkers," as they were called, who cared for little else besides our rupees. This girl emulated the dignity of one born to nobility rather than peasantry. She neither accosted us with beggary nor imposed on us with pride.

In the Strawberry theme, we find one who owns a kingly spirit and can play even the role of beggar or servant with the graciousness befitting nobility. These individuals emote a certain regality of posture. Their very pose says, "I deserve to carry myself upright." Graceful in their body language, their gestures tend to be grand but also quiet—unlike Pineapple themes who can be grandiose, indeed, but minus Strawberry's poise. And what makes Strawberry themes so beautiful? Their ability to see beauty everywhere—in everything and everyone, including themselves.

An interesting keynote of Strawberry themes is that the women tend to be very feminine and the men notably masculine—not to be confused with macho—in ways that communicate the higher octave of their gender. Designers, artisans, ballet dancers, and opera stars—these connoisseurs of beauty are all illustrative of the Strawberry theme. These people also make very healing companions. Their quiet bearing reminds us that we are all deserving of life's riches.

FAMOUS THEME PERSONALITIES

> Sophia Loren
> Grace Kelly
> Rudolph Valentino
> Jacqueline Onassis
> Fred Astaire
> Princess Di
> The Ugly Duckling
> Lady (of Lady and The Tramp)
> Princess in *The Princess and The Pea*
> Amelita Galli-Curci

Not all Strawberry themes are physically beautiful but, at the same time, the quality of dignity beautifies them. Sophia Loren is our classic and classy rags-to-riches Strawberry theme profile. This "Napolitana," born Sophia Scicolone in a ward for unwed mothers eventually married a multi-millionaire. More importantly, through commitment and hard work, she became one of the greatest Strawberry themes ever to grace the movie screens. Ms. Loren shares in her autobiography that she never sells herself short or judges herself by the standards of others. Adhering to high ideals, she claims full responsibility for her successes and failures alike.

All too often, the aging process robs people of their physical beauty and reveals beneath it the "meannesses of the heart," as they are called in yogic teachings. Ms. Loren defines age, simply, as how you feel about yourself. Although now in her senior years, this Strawberry theme has grown more stunning over time. "I'm convinced that outward beauty is directly connected with inward beauty," she relates. "Eyes are not beautiful simply because they are big and wide set, but also because they express something that radiates from the inner woman. My eyes are a precise mirror of my soul."[13] The timeless beauty of Ms. Loren's dedication to ennobling qualities honorably represents her as a true Strawberry theme.

CONFESSIONS OF A STRAWBERRY THEME: LINDA'S TALE

"My childhood was a different one because I was born in Australia and we traveled around a great deal. When I was six, we went to Burma for three years, then America for a year, and Singapore for three years. My father was an international air conditioner salesman. He was Australian and my mother was American. I had a sort of ambivalent upbringing. I don't think my home life was particularly good or bad. My father had problems with drinking, although he maintained a job his whole life. My early years were ones of cocktail parties and servants.

"My strengths? I think I'm a loyal friend, a good mother, a good wife. Being a good mother means that you simply want to *be* a good mother. You can't ever really know what the other person truly needs—you can just try to be there as much as you can to the degree you're able to perceive their needs. I think to some degree I am probably over-responsible. I try too hard to meet other people's needs. Guilt too is an issue for me—not feeling good enough, not feeling worthy.

"Yes, I would say I have lots of dignity. I have an awareness of what dignity is—being centered in oneself. There's an aspect of behavioral awareness. I was raised more by my father who had the British sense of proper behavior—'this is done and this isn't done' sort of thing. I think that contributes to a sort of social self-control and sense of dignity.

"I like strawberries, though I wouldn't say I adore them. But on the other hand, one doesn't get good strawberries any more. Those you get in the stores are just sort of sour or watery, so I have only a vague recollection of really sweet strawberries. I tried to grow them this summer but didn't succeed very well."

WRAPPING IT UP

Quiet dignity springs from deep self-knowledge. Strawberry allows us to honor our true worth and inner strength. Its pervasive quietude springs from a sense of acceptance that life has given to, and taken from, us according to our own role in the grander scheme of things. Whatever now is, simply is. The little Strawberry Essence's quality of self-acceptance becomes Self-acceptance. As rightful kings and queens, we sit on the throne of our own divinity.

STRAWBERRY	*Contrasted With:*	*Companioned With:*
Banana	quiet dignity through humility	for seeing dysfunction as a part of the process toward integration as lessons are learned
Peach	for stable and clear-flowing energy	for integrity developed through the act of giving; conscious mothering with healthy boundaries
Pineapple	well-developed sense of self and healthy, confident self-image	for strength of character and a well integrated, functional personality

POSITIVE EXPRESSIONS

Dignified	Regal bearing
Self-worthiness	Refined tastes
Decisive	Practical
Dependable	Committed
Solid	Loving of beauty
Mature	Integritous
Quiet	Healthy body image
Unassuming	Elegant
Speaks little	Self-respecting

NEGATIVE CONDITIONS

Shy	Spacey
Guilt-ridden	Psychically oversensitive
Poor self-image	"Psychic sponge"
Lacking in self-worth	Dealing with a break-up
Uncentered	Overconscientious
Irresponsible	Clumsy
Feeling lost	Overly apologetic
Uprooted	Ambivalent
Insecure	Indecisive
Relationship difficulties	Feeling inadequate
Self-blaming	Comparing self to others
Abandonment issues	Fearful of aging
Proud	

ESSENCE ENHANCERS

Go to the opera, symphony, ballet, or theater.

Go shopping. Buy yourself something special that says "you are worth it."

Treat yourself to a special meal out.

Pay attention to your posture. Especially keep your shoulders back No slumping!

Identify with your strengths, your talents, your special brand of goodness—and even more to your soul's beauty. Do not allow yourself to fall prey to self-deprecating thoughts.

VISUALIZATION

Close your eyes. Focus on your breathing. Imagine that each inhalation makes you slightly taller and more majestic in spirit. With each exhalation, relax the muscles of your face more deeply. Bring the focus of your attention, drawn through the act of smiling and relaxing the muscles around your eyes, to the point between and just above your eyebrows. The purpose of fixity at this point is to uplift you, to free you from all the mental chains that have weighted you down in your waking existence. Imagine now in some detail, that all sense of unworthiness, imperfection, and lack fall away from you with each ensuing breath.

You are floating, floating in space, wafting upward on clouds of comfort, clouds of contentment. A deep sense of fulfillment—the riches of kings, queens and empires—permeates the temple of your body, your mind, and your spirit. These are the riches of royalty—only they are not counted in gold coins and material trinkets. Yours are the riches of character, full to overflowing with noble qualities gathered over many years—worthwhile years, happy years, ennobling years.

Return now to the welcome friend of each breath. When you are ready, open your eyes and silently repeat the following affirmation.

AFFIRMATION

I am strong in myself, for I am one with what IS!

Rubus strigosus
("prickly, stiff-bristled berry")

CHAPTER TWENTY-EIGHT

RASPBERRY:
"THE HEALER'S HEALER"

"I wanted to be able to let go and forgive a former boyfriend. This took place on Raspberry. I wanted to let go of blaming my daughter, to forgive her and myself for things that had happened between us. On Raspberry, a real shift took place within me and my attitude towards Juliette has changed. I feel that the hurt has healed."

—CNF, Palo Alto, CA

"My chiropractor muscle-tested me for Spirit-in-Nature. Raspberry came up really strongly. He called me a 'tough nut to crack.' I took it for a week and was able to see that I had been thinking only of myself in many of my relationships." —JP, Los Angeles, CA

"I work with people a lot and will periodically do month-long programs. I was concerned about not losing the connection with my students. Raspberry helped me stay connected." —JV, Nevada City, CA

"Taking Raspberry for a week got me thinking about how I treat others in relationships. My response to this essence was very strong."

—JP, Ventura, CA

"My twenty-one-year-old daughter noticed a nice difference in me on Raspberry and wondered what had gotten into me!"

—CL, Cottage Grove, OR

237

"Kindness in words creates confidence. Kindness in thinking creates profoundness. Kindness in giving creates love."   —Lao-tzu

FLOWER/FRUIT/FOLKLORE

This hardy species of the rose family was first cultivated four hundred years ago in Europe and now grows wild in Britain and much of the Northern hemisphere. The Cherokee Indians made much use of the purple variety. From the tiny white flowers on the thorny stems of this bramble fruit, upright canes grow and produce berries. Raspberries are a good source of vitamins A and C. They are an excellent cleanser for mucus, catarrhal conditions, and for toxins in the body. Raspberry leaf tea is a superior female tonic, especially for pregnancy as well as painful menstruation.

Qualities: Kindness, Compassion
Message of Self-mastery: Forgiveness; sympathy; taking responsibility for one's actions; benevolence; generosity; for releasing old wounds; desire to help others; the ability to "turn the other cheek."
Pattern of Disharmony: Feelings easily hurt; a touchy nature; for taking things too personally; for when people say hurtful things; over-reactiveness; insensitivity; for lashing out; lacking understanding; blaming others; resentment; bitterness; attitude of "I don't deserve this"; unkindness.

SPECTRUM PLACEMENT

Quadrant IV's fourth house marks the turning point from Strawberry's sense of self-worth to Raspberry's heightened sensitivity to others. It is the house of kindness, forgiveness, and compassion. Called the "healer's essence," Raspberry combines the feminine quality of the heart's intuition with the finely aged wisdom that is characteristic of this last Quadrant. It is an apt transitional essence for Grape, being expansively loving and profoundly caring.

POSITIVE APPLICATIONS

Raspberry could be called the essence for our age, with its feminine gentleness and compassionate nurturing so needed in these troubled times. One in the positive Raspberry state can be both forgiving and compassionate. Similar to other Quadrant IV essences, positive Raspberry reflects our understanding that the hurts that come to us are our teachers. Our lesson is to reciprocate only love when others treat us poorly. Our task is not to retaliate, but rather to deflect their unkindness and thus be freed of any emotional thorns of inner conflict.

Those who have learned this lesson of Raspberry make excellent teachers, counselors, and therapists. These individuals qualify for any occupation that involves working closely with others, for they have mastered the ability to transmute negative and harmful emotions. To hold a grudge does far more damage to the holder than the individual at whom it is directed. Grudges are like bricks—one by one, they create an entire wall of resentment, preventing a forward movement of energy. Grudges leave one heavy-hearted, even hard-hearted, instead of the desired opposite—kindhearted.

The positive Raspberry state acts as a vibrational salve for the wounds of the heart. The healing professions abound with individuals strong in Raspberry-like qualities, simply because their own past pains have taught them great compassion. Sympathizing, empathizing, and listening are their hallmarks. Lastly, please know that you needn't be emotionally wounded to take Raspberry. It also helps kind people to be even kinder!

NEGATIVE INDICATIONS

The negative Raspberry condition is present in those who are easily hurt; who react emotionally; who lash out without apparent reason; or who are just plain "not nice." All of these actions can indicate either an immaturity, in the sense of not yet having matured, or an aftershock to an emotional wound not yet healed. Men more often than women tend to express this angry/hurt pattern because our culture does not allow them to openly show their feelings. Those who do so may find themselves objects of ridicule that only serves to further suppress their true feelings.

If Raspberry is the essence for forgiveness, then the negative Raspberry state is one of bitterness, resentment, and blaming others. Administering this essence will either allow the issue in question to dissolve or to be talked out until the emotional climate is cleared.

Raspberry is the essence for partners in relationships that terminate without satisfactory reconciliation. When dear friendships end on a bitter note, Raspberry is indicated. For long-term relationships ending in separation with no friendship salvaged, this essence is once again recommended. When marriages dissolve into ugly court battles or lingering animosities, again, look to Raspberry. Sadly, ours is a culture rent with divorce, although there are cases in which no other solution is possible. Especially if children are involved, Raspberry helps to initiate a peaceable friendship and thereby minimize the emotional scarring for all involved.

THEME CHARACTERISTICS

The physical characteristics of the Raspberry theme are subtle. Similar but not identical to Date's softness around the eyes, Raspberry theme energy is detectable as a gentleness *in* the eyes. Looking into the eyes of a Raspberry theme will make you want to pour out your heart. The unspoken message is, "I am here for you. Please share anything that will help you to make peace with yourself." A Raspberry theme is trusting, trustworthy, and "safe" to talk to. Look for those rosy Raspberry cheeks so characteristic of this theme.

You will not find many Raspberry themes in the public eye, but rather administering loving support behind the scenes. These are the quiet cheerleaders, and champions of humanity—the counselors, teachers and volunteer workers. Like Banana themes, they make wonderful listeners. Similar to Almond themes, they remain inconspicuous and tend to pass unnoticed through life's maddening crowds. You could say that Raspberry themes are "all heart"—and the heart at its best excels in the quality of loving receptivity.

Interestingly, in the context of food combining, raspberries are the only fruit that can be eaten with either acidic or alkaline foods. Metaphorically speaking, the Raspberry theme being self-forgiving and forgiving of others, can move through life quietly, able to mix with many different personality types.

FAMOUS THEME PERSONALITIES

Forrest Gump

Dr. Edward Bach

Joseph Cornell

Anne Frank

Maria Montessori

Oprah Winfrey

Carrie Chapman Catt

Edgar Cayce

Corrie Ten Boom

"I'm not a smart man, but I know what love is." With these words, Forrest Gump—the film's star and namesake—quietly accepted his sweetheart's marriage proposal rejection. He harbors no bitterness and no need to retaliate. There is only his straight-from-the-heart Raspberry theme confession. The movie, *Forrest Gump*, spans three decades of American history. From polio survivor to football legend, from Vietnam war medals to White House honors, Mr. Gump became the world's most unassuming "godzillionaire." He used the resources of his heart and his wallet to enrich the lives of those around him.

Polio confined the young Forrest to leg braces. In one of the film's more powerful scenes, we see a slow-motion close-up of his legs. As he begins to "run like the wind blows," Forrest breaks free of his braces, and of the delusion of physical frailty. Ironically, he finds himself chased by bullies in this scene, for whom he harbors no ill will. The young Forrest, caring to a fault, expresses the depth of Raspberry's forgiveness by returning only love to his aggressors—his unkind schoolmates, a bitter lieutenant, and the woman who scorns him for many years.

Lest we be tempted to label Forrest as a Spinach theme merely on the basis of a below-average IQ, a Spinach sub-theme is more accurate for the positive qualities of his childlike nature. Set in a time of our country's rebellious hippie drug years, Forrest's Spinach-like innocence and trust of people's innate goodness inspire us. An accusatory, sarcastic Lieutenant Dan who lost both legs in the war—and a perfect example of the negative Raspberry state—barks, "Gump, have you found Jesus yet?" With Spinach-like simplicity, Forrest responds, "I didn't know I was supposed to be lookin' for 'im."

CONFESSIONS OF A RASPBERRY THEME: IN DENICE'S WORDS

"I love being around people. I really enjoy one-on-one interactions, and I like in-depth conversations. I'm not really good at small talk, nor do I enjoy it. I never know what to say in small talk! There's just so much else to say, I feel really foolish. I'd just rather go to the heart.

"Qualities I most admire in others? There are so many! I especially admire those who share unconditional love and are non-judgmental and open-hearted, and balanced with head and heart. I really value the heart qualities. Now that I think about it, I have tremendous respect for people who have a lot of heart but are also clear thinkers and practical.

"I'm certainly striving to be kind-hearted. I feel like my mother is the epitome of kind-hearted—just so loving and giving to others. I think it's something to aspire to. I don't know that I've reached it. It's my ideal, though I feel I've fallen short of it.

"My feelings are easily hurt, and I have to work at not taking things so personally. Right now, I'm doing a lot of introspection. I'm working now on releasing old wounds. I feel like God said, 'I'm going to give you an incredible home and life in which to release all your old pain.' I was saying to my husband today that I feel like I should be an old, wise woman. That's really what I want to be—kind of a feminine nurturer as the crone figure who can help others because she's experienced it or just because she knows.

"I *love* raspberries! Making raspberry jam—giving it away as presents in those wonderful little jars at Christmastime. It's my favorite icing on chocolate cake. I don't do chocolate icing on chocolate cake, only raspberries on top!"

WRAPPING IT UP

There is a true story of a rabbi who lost his entire family—wife, child, and parents—in the Holocaust. Epitomizing the positive Raspberry state, he chose forgiveness over bitterness and resentment. Why? He said he did not want to bring Hitler along with him when he relocated to America.

Forgiveness heals the body as well as the heart. The contrary is also true. Studies have shown that reliving past hurts over and over again is physically harmful and that the mere memory of an unresolved bitter incident is stressful to the heart. Lingering grudges have been linked to coronary artery disease, high blood pressure, and lowered immunity to other diseases.

Raspberry, then, is a vital essence for emotional well-being. In choosing to let go of past hurts, we embrace health. As Confucius reminds us, "To be wronged is nothing unless you remember it." In taking responsibility for our actions—being loving instead of nursing hurts—we become whole in ways that allow us to in turn help others in their quest for wholeness. Raspberry is the healer of hurts; the comforter of pain; the balm for the wounded warrior who refuses to exit the battlefield until he has conquered every obstacle to his goal—the ability to love perfectly.

RASPBERRY	*Contrasted With:*	*Companioned With:*
Cherry	for lightheartedness	to balance lightness with depth of insight
Grape	for relating to others without expectation or need	for a heart that is both open and fearless
Peach	for compassion, caring deeply for others	for "being there" for those in need

POSITIVE EXPRESSIONS

Kind-hearted
Able to let go
Sympathetic
Benevolent
Empathetic
Compassionate
Loving

Forgiving
Generous
Able to release hurts
Understanding
Wise
Good listener

NEGATIVE CONDITIONS

Bitter
Resentful
Easily hurt
Over-reactive
Insensitive to others
Blaming of others
Touchy

Holding grudges
Mean
Cruel
Nasty
Unkind
Lashing out
Overly emotional

ESSENCE ENHANCERS

Develop existing friendships. Call a good friend and try to be a listener.

If you have any friendships or relationships that have ended bitterly or are unresolved, patch them up. If this is not possible due to death or their unwillingness, work with prayer to reach a resolution within yourself. Other options are: a self-help book or prayer.

Repeat the following visualization until you feel the relationship in question is cleared of all negativity.

VISUALIZATION

Sit quietly in a comfortable place.

With closed eyes, focus your attention at your heart center—not the physical organ but the center of your astral spine that both gives and receives love. The physical heart is finite; the heart's spirit is infinite. Feel the boundaries of your heart expanding. Identify yourself with that boundless expanse of space. Now draw to mind friends and family members whom you love. Perhaps some have passed on or moved away. Let not time or distance impede the flow of kindly, loving thoughts to them.

Imagine these dear people, one by one, as children. One at a time, reach down and take each one's hand as you walk through a flowered mountain meadow together. Feel a current of love coursing from your heart through your arm, and out your palm into theirs.

Hold this image of walking through a meadow. This time, though, the person's hand in yours belongs to someone who has deeply hurt you. Resist the instinctive, self-protective desire to withdraw your hand. Deliberately and consciously extend a flow of heart energy to this special person. Rather than focusing on the details of what needs to be forgiven and whatever sharp thread of bitterness that remains, concentrate on sending love.

Let these waves of love blend with the delicate aroma of the wild-flowers and the cool mountain breeze. To give love to those dear to you is kindly; to return only loving kindness to those who have hurt you is heroic.

AFFIRMATION

In kindness I am one with all. The perfume of unconditional love blows through me to touch their hearts.

CHAPTER TWENTY-NINE

GRAPE:
"THE REWARDER"

Vitis vinifera
("cultivated wine grape")

"I was already drinking grape juice like crazy, so I decided to take the essence. I immediately felt calm and loving, sort of an inner smile. It seemed on Grape that people just wanted my energy. The eighteen-year-old daughter of a friend asked me to hug her, and a whole family in a restaurant came up and started talking to me in detail! I was on vacation and it was a calm and loving trip for both my husband and me."
— *JS, Plano, TX*

"I was lonely, overwhelmed, severely stressed and burnt out as a single mother. Plus, I had this ugly boil on my face and was very self-conscious that brought up a lot of body-image issues. I woke up the next two mornings after taking Grape and feeling a definite change for the better. I had been so unhappy before!" — *MH, North San Juan, CA*

"Grape helped me with the emotional issues around PMS. I used to chew out my family and have suicidal thoughts. Now I only have two rough hours instead of two weeks to deal with each month."
— *SVC, Nevada City, CA*

"This one (Grape) helped me to know who I was. I've had to deal with the reality of not being close to my husband. On Grape, I felt light and was hugging myself." — *UK, Salt Lake City, UT*

"Grape helped me within one week. I started writing poetry. I've never been able to do that before! It felt like it opened my heart. I'd be driving around and verses would come to me, first in the form of prose, so I started writing them down. When I went off Grape, the poetry stopped— so I'm thinking of taking it again." —*BM, Dallas, TX*

"I'd been wanting a relationship for some time. I met a woman and had a lovely romance the night I started Grape. That doesn't happen to me often!"
— *RR, Pahoa, HI*

"Love is a fruit in season at all times." —Mother Teresa

FLOWER/FRUIT/FOLKLORE

One of the oldest cultivated fruits in history, grapes were grown by the ancient Egyptians about six thousand years ago. These thornless vines climb by tendrils and produce tiny greenish flowers in clusters. Roughly six to eight thousand different varieties have been identified. Grapes contain significant amounts of fiber, magnesium, potassium, and vitamins A, B, and C. They are rich in curative properties, and the juice is often used for fasting. Soothing to the nervous system, grapes also assist the bowels, liver, kidneys, and bladder. The darker varieties of grapes are high in iron, making them an excellent blood builder.

Qualities: Love, Devotion
Message of Self-mastery: Realization of the inner source of love; purity; loving without condition, demand, or expectation; patience with others' shortcomings; flowing with the longer rhythms in relationships; healthy sexuality; for transcendence.
Pattern of Disharmony: Negative emotions such as envy, greed, lust, jealousy; for issues of abandonment, including separation, divorce, or death; neediness; cruelty; loneliness; feeling disconnected; feeling alienated; a noncommittal nature; vulnerability; "sour grapes" attitude.

SPECTRUM PLACEMENT

Our journey ends in Quadrant IV's final house with the quality of love. Grape resides at the Spectrum's zenith of the feminine half, for love makes us receptive. We have now observed the inner odyssey through each of the essences, gathering the special gifts of each quality like a bouquet of varied wildflowers. From Raspberry's yearning to aid the healing of a hurting humanity dawns the devotion of Grape's genuine love. Internalizing the lessons of this last house, our quest for wholeness is now complete.

POSITIVE APPLICATIONS

Love is the essence of relationships—with a partner, a child, a parent, a friend, and with ourselves. *We are relational beings.* As the popular song says, we are "people who need people." Although not everyone is cut out for or desirous of a close love relationship, here are some facts to consider:

"Health statistics reveal our innate need for relationship. People who are single over long periods of time tend to suffer from depression to one degree or another; they have weakened immune systems and so are more vulnerable to disease and have a shorter life expectancy. They are also less efficient in the workplace, and less able to weather crisis or disappointment. It is practically commonplace for a widowed person to go into decline, to become ill and even die within a year or so of a spouse's death—whether the marriage was a happy one or not. And numerous studies have demonstrated the withering effect of neglect or lack of affection on babies." [14]

The positive Grape state is one of an open heart, willing to take the risks involved in opening up to others. "I'd rather be hurt a thousand times," said a friend, "than lose the capacity to love." In fact, a common response to Grape is crying, a sign of a closed heart in the process of opening. "I had shut down from past relationship wounds," Chloe confessed to her massage therapist. "I cried a lot for two days on Grape and then felt fine—changed." Phil recounted a similar story: "I cried for three hours a couple of days in a row. I just felt this impersonal sadness about the separation of mankind from its source. As a result of these few days, I now feel a greater awareness. Many insights have come." Laurel's story, too, illustrates how Grape can benefit us in the dance of relationships in which we sometimes, unwittingly and unintentionally, step on our partner's toes:

"Geoff and I are both under much pressure in regard to selling the house and the timing of an interstate move. It brings up a lot of stuff and some of our patterns are as old as our relationship. We fell into one of our patterns of disagreement and, as usual, it felt awful. He yells, I cry. We both seemed to be in that twilight zone place of being misunderstood.

"When he went to work, I put two little Grape drops in a glass of spring water on the counter and sipped it whenever I walked by. I noticed within hours that I was feeling differently than I would have before under similar circumstances. The first word that comes to mind is that there was a 'softening.' Somehow, some of my thoughts loosened up. I didn't feel so heavy-hearted. I had more kind words to offer my two kids. The key here is that, even without further interaction with Geoff, I felt something had been worked out.

"Anyway, I have to tell you—as odd as this seems to put it right out there on paper—there was a point late in the afternoon when, as I mulled over the experience I was having, the words came into my head that. . .I have *become* love. If that isn't a profound moment, I can't imagine what is. Even though I have not sustained the exact feeling of that moment, I still have a sense of it."

The simple message of Grape is unconditional love. "You learn to love by loving," St. Francis of Sales noted. "Begin as a mere apprentice, and the very power of love will lead you on to become a master in the art." And a Jewish saying which humorously illustrates Grape's love coupled with acceptance advises: Love thy neighbor, even when he plays the trombone.

NEGATIVE INDICATIONS

Poets throughout the ages have extolled love's power and beauty. "Take away love and our earth is a tomb," mused Robert Browning. "Man, while he loves, is never quite depraved," philosophized English essayist Charles Lamb. Indeed, we do feel deprived in the negative Grape state. This essence deals directly with those periods when we feel a lack or loss of love in our lives from death, divorce, separation, loneliness, emptiness, or experience feelings of abandonment. Any sense of neediness, isolation, or disconnectedness sounds the warning signal on the negative Grape condition. How do we recognize this state? It just doesn't feel good. Something is missing and that "something" is our choice to be a channel for love.

Grape is the perfect essence for the loss of a loved one. The message of this essence is to look within, and then give to others the very love we feel has been lost.

"It is better to have loved and lost," counsels the poet Tennyson, "than never to have loved at all." If we *have* loved and lost, our natural defense mechanism—and a symptom of the negative Grape state—is to shut down and fabricate barriers to ward off the fear of any future disappointment. Unfortunately, this action only creates more problems.

Love is powerful and its absence in any form can be a major source of suffering. Mother Theresa of Calcutta, who nursed thousands of the homeless, hungry, and ill, once said that she found no suffering greater than the loneliness of people in America's crowded cities. To make matters worse, we are accustomed to looking for sources outside ourselves to heal this deepest of pains. And while relationships are a vital source of connectedness and nurturance, the lesson of Grape is to find that love from within. The best cure for loneliness is to befriend the lonely; the remedy for grief is to comfort the grieving. Life becomes dry without love. Like the grape vine that entwines its leaves around whatever it grows on, it is our nature to develop divine love and devotion.

To live a full life, our heart's feelings must be awakened. Don't wait in the hope that others will love you. Love them spontaneously, whatever their feeling for you! Grape helps to develop selfless love for everyone and everything. Best of all, it helps to develop a love for God and for all true and noble qualities.

THEME CHARACTERISTICS

Grape themes tend to have a roundedness to their appearance. Even if they are not overweight, their presence emits a certain fullness. Oddly enough, you may not be able to recall their physical features in their absence. The reason for this phenomena is simply that it is their spirit which leaves an impression and not their physical attributes. One

Grape theme mentioned that her close friends and family always tell her that she's lost weight—even though it has remained the same since high school—and they invariably buy her clothing at least two sizes too large! Grape themes are very huggable. Their extra-special hugs accompany their approachableness and warmth. In their presence, you will feel childlike, accepted, nurtured and, most of all, inspired by the depth and breadth of their ability—and yours—to love unconditionally.

FAMOUS THEME PERSONALITIES

Padre Pio
Albert Einstein
Norman Rockwell
Paramhansa Yogananda
St. Therese of Lisieux *
Johann Sebastian Bach
Brother Lawrence
St. John of the Cross
Daniel Considine

Our Grape theme is personified by an obscure Italian priest, Padre Pio, who bore the stigmata on his hands and feet for the last fifty years of his life. So great was his divine love that his continuously bleeding wounds, although a source of unrelenting pain, barely distracted him. Before his passing in 1968 at the age of eighty-one, thousands came to take confession from him and hear his 5 a.m. mass that often lasted hours instead of the traditional twenty minutes. Scores of crowds witnessed his utter absorption in a depthless devotion and thereby found that same source of unconditional love awakened within their own receptive hearts.

The Capuchin priest describes his inner life in these words: "I no sooner begin to pray than my heart becomes filled with a fire of love; this fire does not resemble any fire of this lowly earth. It is a sweet and delicate flame which consumes yet causes no pain. It is so sweet and delicate that it satisfies and satiates my spirit to the point of insatiability."

Many miraculous healings surrounded Padre Pio's simple life. To this day, over a million people visit his tomb each year in the small town of Foggia, their pilgrimages honoring the divine love that poured so effortlessly from his humble spirit.

CONFESSIONS OF A GRAPE THEME: IN CONNIE'S WORDS

(A note here: Our gracious Grape, with a strong Raspberry sub-theme, articulated the spirit of this theme with such insightful clarity that I have taken the liberty of leaving her testimony virtually uncut.)

"I grew up in a very loving family, the third of four children. Middle America, suburban, having all the material things. First color TV on the block, big swimming pool, all the stuff. Everything was right out of Ozzie and Harriet until about puberty when my father started drinking and my mother was probably going through menopause, but nobody ever talked about what was happening if they weren't doing too well. As a result of this time, there are definitely some issues in my life. That was an era when people didn't get counseling. We didn't even *know* people who were divorced. It was the 'nifty fifties.'

"I was a very happy child—I really was. I was outgoing, a full A student, real cute, teacher's pet. It all worked for me. I felt like I had the world by the tail. In adolescence, that all changed because I didn't have a Barbie Doll body. Also, the hippie flower child revolution started happening, and I was searching for meaning. So I went right into that whole drug subculture scene. It felt very meaningful to me, like I was exactly in the right place. I made a great hippie.

"My father was a real lover of nature. So we would leave suburbia and our postage-stamp backyard and go out into the woods of Michigan with the birch trees and the deer. I had a sense from very early on that I related to God in nature. I always drew a lot of inspiration there. I was aware of how wide open, how different I felt in nature. I felt fed. Nature was food to me. Things made sense in nature. You know, it was okay that a tree died because it went back into the earth and recycled itself. It made sense that there was a chain of command in the animal kingdom. But suburbia didn't make sense to me. I didn't want to wear those blouses with bows.

"My official job title? Family counselor. I've got a lot of humor; I spend a lot of time making jokes and lightening up the situation when people are struggling. People tell me I'm a very nurturing individual. I've always felt serviceful. I feel full when I give to other people.

"I would say I am a loving person. I love people, I really do. I feel a lot of unconditional love and compassion for others. I think people feel safe with me. They can tell me yucky things about themselves and know that I will still be their friend and keep confidences about issues that they have. I think devotion is my path—to perfect that heart quality and to take all the love that I have for people and expand it into seeing that it's God I love in them. I think that's what I'm doing.

"I love my children to the point of attachment. It was very difficult letting go of my oldest child when she went off to college. I went through a real grieving process quite unexpectedly, much deeper and more profound than I thought might happen. It was very expansive for me to let her go out into the world and know I personally wouldn't be able to protect her—and that I had never really been the one doing that anyway. To be able to see that she would be protected by others was big for me.

"I *love* grapes. I have grapes planted all over my yard. I just love grapes, I love grape juice, and used to love wine too. I hang out under the grape arbor. I like to take my journal and sit there on my blanket. We have these beautiful little trellises of grapes. And I love grape leaves, the shape of them. I do a grape juice fast every year when grapes are in season for usually three or four days, fresh and watered down a bit if it's too intense.

"As I was telling you about sitting under the grape vines, I had this memory of going to my grandmother's. She lived out on a lake and her whole yard was bordered by grapes. I remember just being so happy there. We got to make wine. She let us step on the grapes in a little washtub. She made wine every year and it was kind of a big family thing to get together and press the grapes."

WRAPPING IT UP

Grapes are a fruit rich in myth and folklore. The Bible mentions their existence during the lime of Noah. Ancient yogic teachings tell us that grapes, when fermented, carry a vibration of passion instead of pure love. In Omar Khayyam's famous "Rubaiyat," grapes are referred to in four separate quatrains, symbolizing a state of ecstatic love.

And what of the quality of devotion, also encapsulated in Grape? The word *devotion* stems from the Latin root *vovere*, meaning "to vow." When we commit ourselves to the act of loving, that love acquires the quality of devotion. Devotional love is a love beyond change, regardless of the passing of time. Perhaps you have heard this generalization about the sexes when a couple marry—that the woman expects the man to change and the man hopes the woman never will. Both partners here are expressing the need for Grape.

Too often, attachment masquerades as love. The lyrics of current popular songs and also of music throughout the ages glorifies this kind of codependence. "I'm gonna make you love me, oh yes I will," affirms a song of the 1970's. And from an old Irish ballad, "I wish I was in the young man's arms that broke the heart of mine." Self-seeking love is binding; genuine love is liberating. Pure love finds its fulfillment in the simple act of loving.

Grape thereby helps us to remove the veil of emotional poverty that steals over us at times and to heal that dryness of the heart that arises from the many sorrows that life lays at our feet. This essence helps to uncover our heart's natural ability to love and in so doing, to forget ourselves in the process to the point where the lover, the beloved, and the act of loving become as one. Love, "the rewarder," is its own reward.

It is said that at the time of our death, we are met on the other side by an angel who asks of us, simply, "Did you love more each day than the day before?" If we can answer to the affirmative, then we have attained the greatest possible achievement.

GRAPE	Contrasted With:	Companioned With:
Cherry	inner freedom from outer circumstances	for finding fulfillment within ourselves, for a playful, loving nature
Peach	loving from wholeness instead of need	selfless love, loving service
Pear	for the peace acquired through genuine love	for an upward flow of dependable energy; strong, unwavering love
Raspberry	for compassion and deep caring	for a heart that is both open and fearless

POSITIVE EXPRESSIONS

Loving	Reverential
Devotional	Non-possessive
Inspirational	Expansive
Peaceful	Respectful
Feeling nurtured	Friendly
Healthy sexuality	Pure
Steadfast	Unconditionally loving
Courteous	Undemanding
A sharing nature	Loving without expectation
Considerate	Patient
Magnetic	Transcendent
Undemanding	Committed

NEGATIVE CONDITIONS

Overbearing

Expecting obedience

Empty

Lonely

Needy

Clinging

Cruel

Pushy

Frigid

Impotent

Having sexual problems

Demanding

Teasing

Unrealistic in expectations

Aloof

Possessive

Critical

Blaming

Inconsiderate

Envious

Greedy

Lustful

Jealous

Abandonment issues

Separation

Divorce

Grieving the death of loved one

Feeling disconnected

Alienated

Noncommittal

Egoistic

Vulnerable

ESSENCE ENHANCERS

When you're out shopping, dining, in line at the movies, or any-where in public, observe relationships and how people treat each other—mother and child, same-sex peers, older couples, boyfriend and girlfriend. Mentally note the dynamics between people. Do you perceive them as loving? Courteous? Expansive with each other?

Review the relationships in your present life and the quality of love you give to others. Note areas that need improvement and resolve to work on them.

Meditate, ending each session with a focused prayer from your heart to send love out into the world.

Stand in the sunlight, both drawing in and sending out rays of love through all the cells in your body.

Try this cure for loneliness—befriend your own mind. Involve yourself in creative projects. In other words, allow yourself dynamic "alone time."

Buy some flowers for yourself or a loved one.

Take yourself out on a date; enjoy your own company.

VISUALIZATION

Am I dreaming? you ask yourself. This can't be what it's like to pass on. There was no pain, just an effortless wafting into the clouds. These are light clouds—not the clouds of an impending thunderstorm, but the soft, billowy clouds that get whooshed away by the slightest icy breeze on a sunny winter's morning.

You are floating, floating, many pounds lighter than you ever remember being while on earth. You can still speak, but your voice is now only an echo of itself. You can see yourself, though you are now only a translucent shadow. Light, everything is light. And the most wonderful thing is that you have no fear—only a deep peace and an even deeper sense of being cocooned in a very great love.

And you can fly! What fun to look *down* on the mountains! How little they look, how tiny the earth. Your life, from this vantage point, looks like a checkerboard; your most loved friends and family, like chess pieces moving to and fro. The wind, like a warm breath, steals up behind you. It takes shape aurally, forming words. The words come into focus, like tuning in a radio dial.

"Did you learn to love more deeply each day than the day before?" The voice comes from nowhere and everywhere. Just as the thought forms, how to answer—a plane flies overhead. It startles you from your reverie. You awaken from the dream.

AFFIRMATION

By loving all, I become whole. I need nothing, for I am ever one with Spirit!

PART III

CHAPTER THIRTY

MAKING THEM, TAKING THEM

"When I touch that flower, I am not merely touching that flower. I am touching
infinity. That little flower existed long before there were human beings on this
earth. It will continue to exist for thousands, yes, millions of years to come."
—George Washington Carver

CAPTURING THE ESSENCE

Preparing a flower essence is not a mechanical process—it's a magical one. The first thing to prepare is *yourself.* The energy with which
you make flower essences affects the quality of the finished product, as
energy is constantly pouring out of our hands. Be fully in the moment,
completely present, and in a very positive state of mind. You might
want to pause and take several deep breaths before beginning, to
attune yourself with the essence-making process. Also, you may want
to take a flower essence to help clear your energy.

You will want to gather your equipment—a plain, clear crystal
bowl (or glass, to avoid the lead content), pure spring water, and high-
quality brandy as a preservative. (Bottled spring water is fine; distilled
is not. The ionization process used in distillation destroys the water's
life force that is necessary to hold the essence's potency.) Lastly, you'll
need a cloudless, sunny morning. Even one cloud passing over the sun
will break the flow of energy required to draw the life force out of the
blossoms and into the water.

Now, fill the bowl with the spring water. Next, cover your fingers
with a leaf from one of the plants or trees that you have selected so that
you do not directly touch the blossoms. Choose flowers as you would
select fruit at the grocery store—the largest, freshest, and most vibrant
of the group at their peak of bloom. Pick those blossoms that grow

in profusion, selecting only a few from each plant or tree so that the plant's integrity is left intact. Work only with organically grown trees and plants whose natural growth is as undisturbed as possible.

Completely cover the surface of the water with the plucked flowers. Set the bowl in a spot where no shadows, including your own, will pass over it for the next three to four hours. At the end of that time, you will see that a magical transformation has taken place—the life force of the blossoms has been infused into the water through the magnetic energy of the sun.

Then, carefully skim off the blossoms with a leaf from the plant and pour the *Mother Essence,* as it is called, into an unused dark glass bottle. If you want to ensure that no blossoms will slip into the bottle, you can pour the Mother Essence through an organic coffee filter. Fill the bottle only halfway with the essence and the remainder with brandy. The brandy serves two purposes: (1) it is a chemical preservative; and (2) it is considered to be an "anchor" to hold the subtle essence vibrations in the water.

The above procedure is called the Sun Method of preparation. Should several hours of unbroken sunlight be unavailable, use the Boiling Method instead. Pick the blossoms in full sunlight in the morning. In a new and unused enamel pot, bring them to a boil in pure spring water. Then, lower the heat to simmer for thirty minutes. Add brandy and store this Mother Essence as explained above. (Note: both the bowl and the pot may be reused for essence preparation after being rinsed with warm sea-salt water. This prevents "vibrational contamination" from previous usage.)

PRESERVING AND STORING THE ESSENCES

To prepare a Stock Concentrate, place two drops of Mother Essence in a one-ounce dark-glass bottle with a glass dropper, and fill the remainder of the bottle with half brandy and half spring water. Once the essence is made, keep it out of sunlight. Mother Essence, Stock Concentrate and Dosage Bottles should be stored in a cool, dark, dry place. Plastic droppers tend to react with the brandy and create an unpleasant taste, so glass is highly preferred.

The Mother Essence is not taken directly, but you may take the Stock Concentrate undiluted—two to four drops, four times a day, under the tongue—or use it to prepare a Dosage Bottle. Practitioners, and those wanting the Stock Concentrate to last longer, can take the time to prepare the Dosage Bottle. This requires adding two drops of Stock Concentrate to a one-ounce dark-glass dropper bottle, one tablespoon of brandy and then filling the bottle with spring water. The essences in Dosage Bottle strength are taken four drops, four times a day. Both the Stock Concentrate and Dosage Bottle essences may be added to water, juice, or tea and sipped throughout the day. If flower essences are properly and hygienically prepared as described above, they will retain their potency for at least six to ten years.

HELPFUL HINTS

For brandy sensitivity—a consideration for many people, including recovering alcoholics, children, and those with candida or other health issues—the brandy may be eliminated from the Dosage Bottle if it is refrigerated. The bottle will retain its potency for a month's time. Or, both Stock and Dosage preparations may be added to a boiling beverage so that the alcohol content evaporates. As an alternative to ingestion, several drops may be placed on the underside of one wrist and rubbed into the other, much like applying perfume.

The creative usage of flower essences is infinitely varied. Here are a few suggestions. Try two Stock drops to one quarter-cup massage oil or body lotion; four Stock drops in a misting bottle to spray exposed parts of the body; or sixteen Stock drops per tub of bath water. For emergencies and also less urgent circumstances, apply the drops directly to the skin, especially on areas in particular need, and rub in the essence. Also, four Stock drops to baby's bottle is a wonderful way to give it to children. A nursing mother can take her baby's essence so that he can receive it through her milk. (This concept applies to animals as well. See Chapter Thirty-five for further directions and Chapter Thirty-four, for children.) Add a couple of drops to fruit pop-sicles of the same essence. Place on acupressure points; acupuncturists may apply Stock to the meridians. Feel free to be adventurous and explore new possibilities for taking the essences. One man shared that he liked to sleep with his Stock bottle under his pillow just to have it close by!

Unlike homeopathy, flower essences are not antidoted by the use of coffee, black tea, chocolate, mint, or other strong spices. Also, there are no determined levels of potency such as 6x, 12x, or 30x. Stock and Dosage preparations are reported by people to be equally as potent in their respective dosage amounts.

Often with allopathic medicines, we read of contra-indications and possible side effects. This is not a concern with flower essences. They readily enhance and supplement other medications, herbs, therapies, and treatments.

Taking the essences more than the minimum suggested dosage of four times daily is helpful—ten or even twenty times, especially in an emergency situation. Although exceeding the dosage *quantity* is not helpful, neither is it harmful. However, other flower essence companies and practitioners vary somewhat in their recommended dosages—two to four Stock drops at a time, though, is quite within the realm of reasonable. If we remember that we're working with vibrational remedies and not biochemical medications, the quantities are less important than taking the essence several times throughout the day. Here's what worked for Renee:

"I could give you this Apple testimonial because I had this cold—no, seriously—I had been suffering with this little cold. It just kept dragging on, and I was taking all kinds of stuff like echinacea, and it wasn't going away. I didn't take Apple the way you're supposed to—I squeezed, like, a whole dropper. I stuck it in my mouth, I mean the whole dropperful every two hours, and my cold was gone the next day. I mean, it was like taking an industrial dose."

Here's a word of caution, however, about wasting your essence bottle, either Stock or Dosage: don't bother trying to overdose. Flower essences are abuse-proof. Their purity makes it impossible. The essences contain an "innate safety valve" so that taking more than the recommended dosage only wastes them. A mother once called in a panic because her son had swallowed an entire Dosage Bottle of Grape. "Does he need to be rushed to the hospital?" she asked frantically. "No," I told her, "there's no problem at all. But you'll need to replace his bottle."

Often—in fact, too often to ignore—people say that they smell or taste the corresponding fruit or vegetable. This can indicate that the smell and taste of the *vibration* of the corresponding food source may be imprinted into the essence itself.

ONE VERSUS MANY

How many essences can we reasonably take at one time? You will find many responses to this question, as varied as the practitioners working with them. Some say nine, others recommend one. It can be argued that we're working on many issues at one time. If we view essences as "bottled affirmations," it is best to focus on one at a time, to "energetically sink our teeth into it," so to speak. This is similar to the homeopathic concept of a single constitutional remedy.

In researching Spirit-in-Nature Essences for nearly forty years, I first worked with combined essences for several years and have since suggested only one at a time. Why one at a time? Each essence is a complete adventure in itself, reaching far beyond the one quality associated with it. Banana for humility also addresses issues of calmness, nonidentification, non-attachment, gentleness and strength. When we take only one essence at a time, we are better able to: (1) isolate which essence is working for us; (2) observe results more quickly, and more dramatically; and (3) focus on that particular essence and its corresponding qualities. People still receive their five essences per month, but sequentially instead of simultaneously. (See Chapter Thirty-three.)

Karen is a case in point. We met several years back in her small health food store. It had been a harried day, she admitted. We spoke briefly, and I left a bottle of Tomato, for strength and courage. She called back three days later with the following testimonial:

"The Tomato took away my PMS in two hours—and it wasn't time for it to be over. I took the essence frequently. Yes, I felt courage or a warrior's spirit. I also felt healed in my heart on the subject of animal cruelty. This is an issue for me, since I always take in stray animals. I also now feel I can do my work more clearly, and I am less influenced by all the different energies one encounters in dealing with the public. I have tried for years through nutrition, herbs, and supplements to achieve what happened overnight with Tomato. My thinking has cleared and my dreams have changed—more color and texture now. Also, even though I am remarried, I feel I have cleared some residual issues from my divorce eighteen years ago."

Oftentimes, as in Karen's case, a single essence will dissolve lingering subconscious issues that we are unaware of. Much like getting a massage that smooths out knotted muscles, we may suddenly realize how much tension we'd been carrying around without even knowing it until, by contrast, the knots were released. Flower essences dissolve psycho-emotional tension in a similar fashion.

The single-essence method raises a certain paradox. While you may take an essence to both support and enhance other supplements and therapies, taking an essence *with other essences* seems to weaken their results, even if only slightly, according to a significant number of my clients' responses. Why? To some extent, they cancel each other out. Would you, for example, go to several acupuncturists or psychotherapists during the same time period? So, consider: *one essence at a time, per person,* rather than one essence per issue.

To clarify: taking one essence at a time doesn't mean that we are only working on one part of our lives at that time. Not at all! Here's an analogy: would you like to listen to five radio stations at once? Clearly, one is enough. The good news is that people tend to progress through their essences more quickly when taking only one at a time. Three days to two weeks is a standard length of time on a remedy in a particular essence cycle. We may choose to return to that essence at a later date, having worked through one level of a given test to our satisfaction. Insights come quickly and change can happen fast. Of course, there are exceptions. Frank, for instance, enthusiastically remained on Cherry for six months, to deal with a particularly difficult divorce where children and many complicated emotional issues, were involved.

WHEN TO START AND WHEN TO STOP

"Oh, rats, I forgot my Pear," said a clerk in the cosmetic section of a busy health food store. How did she know she needed an essence? She just did. Experience had taught her that on busier days, Pear was "just what the doctor ordered" to help her deal with the crowds, the questions, and the craziness.

Other indications that it is time to begin an essence are:

You feel the lack of a certain quality in your life—an absence of clarity when decisions need to be made (Blackberry or Avocado), or intolerance when the in-laws pay a visit (Date or possibly Lettuce). NOTE: See Chapter Eight for plot essences.

Things are going well but you have a sense that they could go even better— you won second place in the local bake sale, cooking being a favorite way of nurturing your family and friends (Peach), or you've just given an excellent lecture at the PTA but felt that you could have surpassed even your own expectations (Pineapple). NOTE: See the theme essence section of Chapter Eight.

Other people comment on what they think you need for self-growth. Although it may not be easy, hear them out—and consider taking Banana to improve your listening skills!

Any time of change. All too often we resist change because it may seem frightening, threatening, or overwhelming. These times, though, are fantastic opportunities for inner growth, Corn being especially helpful, although other essences may also be useful.

You find yourself drawn to a particular food, even craving it, and eating more of it than usual. Conversely, you might find yourself repelled by that food, having previously enjoyed it. This can be a way of saying, "I don't want to grow *that* much." In either case, try taking the corresponding essence and see what happens.

You want to learn more about them. We make very suitable guinea pigs for testing out the flower essences. Through our own direct experience in taking them, they open the door to our ability to work successfully with others.

How will you know when you've finished with an essence? See if you feel comfortably stabilized in the changes it effected. That will be a good time to stop and either begin another essence, or remain "essenceless" for awhile. Remember that flower essences are "pump primers"—there is no need to take them indefinitely or for long periods of time.

One invariably accurate clue as to when you have completed an essence is simply this: you begin forgetting to take it. When something is helpful to us, we want it. Trusting our intuition is important. However, forgetting to take a remedy from Day One of an essence program is a different issue—negligence.

WHEN THE REMEDIES DON'T WORK

There are times when we experience no discernible results from taking the essences. The following points can explain why:

Irregularity: I have learned to ask point blank when a client volunteers the no-results feedback, how many times a day he is taking the essence. Nine times out of ten, the answer is, once or twice. The essences must be taken as directed to be effective. They need to be re-introduced into our energy field *at least* four times a day.

The "wrong" essence: Although in truth there are no wrong essences, there are "better" and "best" choices. Use your judgment combined with intuition in assessing immediate needs. Remember to trust yourself. If you don't experience at least the beginning of results within three days, move on to your "next best" choice.

Timing: If you have just begun a new exercise regime, seriously cleaned up your diet, or started on supplements and herbal teas all at one time, you may simply be on overload. It's best to wait until you have integrated your new routine and then, when you can give it your focused attention, begin a program of flower essences.

Lack of need: Just as we don't need to change the oil in our car constantly, we will find times in our lives when we simply don't need to take essences. When our inner machinery is well enough oiled with energy, insight, and peace—these are the times to work with the positive momentum generated by the essences and our willingness to grow. Enjoy these times!

Sometimes the ego resists change: In every moment of our lives, we have the same choice—to move toward the light or away from it. At times, we may simply choose to resist our own growth; the essences won't override your decision.

Dark night: Haven't we all experienced times of suffering so profound that it seems as if no other human being has ever known such anguish? Various religions refer to this time as the "dark night of the soul." This is a state of utter despair in which all outer methods of assistance, including flower essences, seem to fail us. What can you do? Meditation, prayer, and patience are time-honored healers. Perhaps you can draw some measure of solace and hope from the following inspirational quotes:

> *"The diamond cannot be polished without friction, nor the man perfected without trials."*   —Chinese proverb

> *"When the heart weeps for what it has lost, the spirit laughs far what it has found."*   —Sufi saying

> *"Love bears all things, believes all things . . . endures all things. Love never ends. "*   —St. Paul

> *"As to me I know of nothing else but miracles."*
>   —Walt Whitman

BOTTLED AFFIRMATIONS

As mentioned previously, we may liken flower essences—pure vibrational examples of exalted qualities—to "bottled affirmations." The scientific term for affirmations is *autogenic training*. The best times to practice them are upon falling asleep or awakening. These specific times are known as hypnogogic states. Thus, immediately before sleep and upon arising—including nap time—are the most beneficial times to repeat affirmations—*and* to take flower remedies. These are the periods when we can most easily penetrate the realm of superconsciousness, also called the Higher Self, that place within us where true inspiration and intuition reside. Or, we might say that these are the times when the door to the subconscious mind stands ajar and the essences are able to penetrate more deeply than during regular waking hours.

Our thoughts both express and mold who we are. Since they have such a powerful effect on our physical bodies, it is paramount to be aware of their content and quality.

Words have power. They can hurt and they can heal. We have all experienced the sting of unkind words and also the joy of being told by someone dear, "I love you." Often, the mind thinks in words. Affirmations are words that we speak to ourselves in an affirmative state of knowing on a deep level that they ring of truth, even if unconfirmed by outer circumstances. As an experiment, repeat the Corn affirmation sometime when you are exhausted: "With boundless energy I rise to greet the world!" Affirmation is not denial. It is, rather, an unwavering declaration of a higher truth—that we are in possession of vast resources of inner vitality, even though our body at that moment may be expressing fatigue.

The best time for affirmations is when taking the corresponding essence. If you find yourself alone, repeat the affirmation aloud with energy, to help it penetrate the subconscious mind. Say it again more softly to the conscious mind and a third time silently, directed toward the superconscious mind.

As with any activity, the more you put into it, the more you will get out of it. Affirmations recycle back to us as much power as we give to them. Said one man, "I don't even take the essences anymore. I just use the affirmations!"

OPTIMUM TIMES TO TAKE FLOWER ESSENCES

Other times to take flower essences for maximum benefit are:

On an empty stomach. Otherwise our life force is diverted by the digestion process. Ten minutes before or one hour after a meal is fine. Before or after meditation. It has been said that meditation happens "when the mind is still and the heart is open"—a perfect time for essence therapy. This is also a wonderful time to feel their effects.

Before, during, or after any type of quiet activity such as walking, yoga postures, light housework, handicrafts, or reading—anything that clears and relaxes the body and mind simultaneously.

Any time the issue arises for which you are taking an essence. (I once took Tomato Essence twenty times in one hour to deal with Los Angeles rush hour traffic on the freeway and then didn't need it for the next two days of driving.)

CHAPTER THIRTY-ONE

Symptom and Core Approaches: A Few Case Studies

"To be or not to be—that is the problem."

—an Italian friend, translating Shakespeare

In mapping out individual essence programs, we may take two
different approaches—*symptom* or *core treatment*—or a combination
of both. Symptom treatment, as its name implies, addresses immediate psycho-emotional issues, *not* physical symptoms. The symptom
approach targets essences for *specific events,* from anything for which
we are prepared to circumstances that take us by surprise. This type of
essence program may be likened to peeling away the petals of a flower
to reach its heart, or core. Core treatment involves working on deeper-
than-surface-layer issues and *specific emotional states.* This approach
directly impacts underlying emotional issues *behind* the events sur-
rounding them.

How do we relate the symptom and core terms to plot and theme
essences? Symptom treatment programs offer peripheral plot essences.
The core approach is comprised of pivotal plot essences, *or* peripheral
plot essences that touch that emotional shades-of-gray area beyond
mere passing need. Theme essences may be recommended in either
core or symptom programs, depending on the assessment of the flower
essence practitioner.

MARK AND DOREEN'S ADVENTURES

Let's look at two consultations that employ the core approach. The first case study also illustrates how flower essences enhance our magnetism as reflected back to us by others. Feedback from people—who are our mirrors, especially in close relationships—is an excellent way to assess our growth through taking the essences.

Mark came for an evening consultation. We spoke at some length about his present situation. He had recently moved to the area and was seeking employment in hotel management. Having had no luck, he was battling the discouragement of one unsuccessful interview after another. For whatever reasons, he had not been drawing the career opportunities in his chosen field for many years, despite a glowing resume. This was not an easy consultation and it required some verbal excavation. "Anything else going on in your life right now that seems important to mention?" I queried. "Not really," he answered thoughtfully, "except that my dad passed away recently after having been in a coma for a few weeks."

Sensing that his unspoken grief over his father's passing had veiled his ability to attract a job, I suggested Grape as the first essence in his program, for bereavement and loss of love. "After taking one stock drop that evening," he reported the next morning, "I felt different, but I didn't know what it was. I've just returned from the grocery store. It was strange, but people were treating me what I would call deference! They were greeting me with esteem, I guess, and looking into my eyes, wanting to make contact. So even though I noticed something last night but couldn't put it into words, I was aware of a change in my magnetism at the store this morning." (Eye contact is a way to both draw and project magnetism.)

Mark's Grape program is an example of core treatment, or the use of essences that address deeper-than-surface issues. We also could have used a symptom approach to his program—Pineapple, for the obvious career and self-worth issues. Instead, I chose Grape for the underlying issue most likely preventing him from successfully landing a job.

In another example of core treatment, I consulted with a gracious spoken woman named Doreen, who asked if there were also essences for her husband. She reported that he verbally abused their oldest daughter, by whom he felt threatened. The daughter, a Peach theme, excelled in sales. Doreen's husband had lost a vice-president position in a previous job. The family now worked together in a successful sporting goods store.

Rather than recommending Grape for abusiveness (symptom treatment), we began his program with Raspberry. I chose this essence for the emotional wounds that he had sustained during childhood, a time in his life when he was made to feel unworthy. Orange followed, for finding enthusiasm within himself so he needn't feel upstaged by his daughter or in competition with her.

Thus, we addressed core issues that ran much deeper than the more obvious, surface-level symptoms. Psycho-emotional symptoms may be treated *per se* by flower essences or viewed as the tip of the iceberg. These symptoms provide clues which lead to more deeply rooted and long-standing issues—in this case, the core issue of the husband's damaged sense of self-worth from childhood.

Lauren and Janine: The Plot Thickens

Only last week, I consulted with Lauren, whose program employs the symptom approach. She had been diagnosed with Chronic Fatigue Syndrome several years earlier. To no avail, she had explored one therapy and supplement after another. Her most troubling symptom was insomnia; a close second was mourning the active, athletic life that she had been forced to relinquish. Exhausted day after day, Lauren found herself in a sort of "quiet, wound-up mental hysteria" at night, unable to obtain needed rest. We talked about Lettuce as a first essence, because it is usually mental restlessness that precludes the physical condition of insomnia. Her report the next morning—she had slept easily and well. Thus, although flower essences do not directly treat physical illness—in Lauren's case the Chronic Fatigue—Lettuce addressed the psycho-emotional issues contributing to the insomnia and nervous exhaustion, making it, by definition, symptom treatment.

We added other essences to complete Lauren's first program—Coconut, for developing a solution-oriented attitude toward the clinical depression caused by the CFS symptoms; Spinach, for grieving over her loss of self, even though not specifically the stage of childhood, and for the ability to trust the process of the illness and its needed lessons; Tomato, for battling food addictions to sweets and coffee as nurturance substitutes; and Raspberry, to resolve the many hurts and hardships resulting from the Chronic Fatigue Syndrome.

Janine's program is another example of the symptom approach, although it also overlaps with some longstanding core issues related to her parents. As we like to see at least three substantiations for each essence that is recommended, Janine explained the issues she was working on at the beginning of our consultation. She said that she felt she needed to forgive her parents, who had both passed away; that, at age sixty, she was looking to return to work; and that she wanted to write children's books for publication.

Raspberry was chosen as the first essence in her program of five. Here was a compassionate woman, still healing from her own childhood wounds while at the same time deeply sensitive to the needs of the children she worked with. (There is a saying that "what is not acknowledged, or healed, persists.")

Her father, at one time a foreman of lemon pickers in Southern California, had been an alcoholic and her mother "relied on prescription drugs to keep herself together." She explained further that at her last two jobs, she didn't have the courage to speak out for herself and was fearful of her boss as an authority figure. Janine profiled several hurtful experiences, warranting Raspberry Essence.

After our consultation as an Essence Enhancer to help release the hurt she had held onto for decades, Janine taped a recording as though speaking directly to each of her parents. She reported back that on Raspberry Essence:

"I felt a little like my old self. While shopping, I heard music being played through the speakers in the store and I felt like dancing. I got some of my spunk back. I noticed I was more talkative and I planted my first garden outside."

The second essence in her program was Orange, to restore a sense of hope and enthusiasm for her future. In the last of her most recent jobs as a social worker in an adoption agency, she had chosen to be fired and was then rehired as a substitute. She described herself like "a deer in the headlights," unable to help the children to be placed in homes that suited their needs. The agency, sad to say, based its matches on finances. Janine felt emotionally drained with no closure with the children and families on leaving the job.

While taking Orange Essence, Janine said that she was finally able to open up to her daughter about her own mother. She continued, "I talked about a lasagna recipe I use that my mother gave me. I found myself singing about joy."

The remainder of her program consisted of Fig, for feeling that she was "between a rock and a hard place" in being unable to deal with difficult coworkers; Peach, to support her mothering nature expressed through her ties with her biological family and with the children she worked with; and Pineapple, specifically for an imminent job interview, saying she didn't think she was assertive enough at work and that this was a part of her problem. (Although she didn't land that particular job, she was kindly told that her resume was very impressive.)

Essence Paths and Programs

We might say that the only difference between symptom and core treatment is one of degree, with symptom treatment addressing more surface-level issues. In consultation, I generally recommend an essence program based on the individual's need to clear and release one level at a time. Thus, each program is determined by: (1) the client's psycho-physiological symptoms; (2) issues which have impacted him since childhood; and (3) an understanding and application of individualized theme and plot essences.

Which approach should you use, then—symptom or core? Both are valid and they are interconnected, providing a framework for understanding essence application. You may want to incorporate these terms in working with yourself, family, friends, and clients.

CHAPTER THIRTY-TWO

SHADOWS ON A SCREEN: MENOPAUSE AND CODEPENDENCE

"The work is easy and the medicine is not far away. If the secret is disclosed, it will be so simple that everyone may get a good laugh."

—Chang Po-Tuan

It's always good to remember that we are not our symptoms, and that we can laugh even in the process of resolving them.

Let's take a look at two current issues and also how to apply flower essences: menopause and codependence. These subjects were selected because (1) both affect great numbers of the population; (2) although menopause is physiologically based, it includes a wide range of emotional symptoms; and (3) conversely, codependence, though primarily a psychological illness, also affects the physical body through increased stress levels, eating disorders and the toll of addictions; and (4) both topics touch the lives of men and women alike—men need to be informed and sensitive to the changes of their partners and friends in menopause ("men, oh, pause!"), and codependence affects practically everyone to some small degree.

TREATING MENOPAUSE WITH FLOWER ESSENCES

Menopause signifies the ending of the menstrual cycle due to decreased levels of estrogen and progesterone. Each year, approximately one and a third million women reach this stage in their lives. Within the next decade, this figure will double. An estimated ten to fifteen percent of menopausal women experience virtually no discomfort; an equal percentage are incapacitated by symptoms (see lists below).

276

Typically beginning between forty-two and fifty-five years of age, many women experience it earlier or go through surgical menopause as a result of hysterectomy. A wide range of treatment options from Hormone Replacement Therapy to Chinese herbs are available. Flower essences also offer a depth of comfort and strength.

PHYSICAL/PSYCHOLOGICAL SYMPTOMS

The range of physiological menopausal symptoms includes:

Changing periods
Excessive bleeding
Heart palpitations
Hot flashes
Urinary incontinence
Frequent urination
Breast tenderness
Skin sensitivities
Brain static
Headaches
Nausea and dizziness
Gastric upset
Aching joints and muscles
Osteoporosis
Greater risk of heart disease
Insomnia
Fatigue
Weight gain
Vaginal dryness
Lowered sex drive

Psycho-emotional symptoms of menopause may be experienced as:

Anxiety
Insecurity
Confusion
Moodiness
Irritability
Anger
Depression
Mental fuzziness
Stress
Disorientation
Memory impairment
Emotional oversensitivity
Paranoia

MENOPAUSE FURTHER DEFINED

Women in menopause experience anywhere from all to none of the above symptoms. Responses to the menopausal years range from, "piece of cake!" to "you'd better have your life together first." Is there life after menopause? Educated women of today now view this important rite of passage as a time of renewed vitality and hope, even referring to hot flashes as "power surges." Our culture, sadly, not only worships the false god of youth, but also tends to revere the graying, balding man over the graciously aging woman. At last, we are beginning to honor the image of the respected tribal crone and her invaluable contribution to society.

To facilitate the changes and challenges of menopause, all twenty flower essences may come into play at one time or another. Here we can see that all of the essences do the same thing in restoring us to a state of balance and that each of the essences may be used for any particular issue. The key to narrowing the selection is to simply tune in to the individual's temperament and most pressing needs in order of importance. Consider the following essence interpretations:

SPIRIT-IN-NATURE ESSENCES APPLIED TO MENOPAUSE

ALMOND   Emotional balance, equilibrium, restoring a sense of proportion.

APPLE   For clarity during changing physical and emotional states.

AVOCADO   For mental sharpness in understanding the menopausal process; for learning its lessons; confusion; disorientation.

BANANA   For nonidentification with menopause-induced changes; for deep calmness and detachment when symptoms interfere with that calmness; knowing that "this too shall pass."

BLACKBERRY   The ability to introspect; to retain a sense of clarity and perspective about symptoms and thus handle them better.

CHERRY   For the lighter emotional symptoms; grumpiness; for hope; for "emotional-roller-coaster days."

COCONUT   The perseverance to "come out the other end," whether "the pause" lasts one year or ten.

CORN   In times of mental fatigue or exhaustion; whenever the need is felt for an "energy treat"; for seeing menopause as a new and exciting stage of life.

DATE   For self-nurturing (fill the bath with sixteen drops of Date Essence and scented herbs—light a candle and incense, and let yourself be nurtured); for judging others; "No one understands me" attitude.

FIG   To relax being too hard on yourself; comparing self to others; thinking you should be doing better than you are.

GRAPE   For love that cures loneliness, isolation; for feeling unloved, especially for taking it out on others (adult temper tantrums).

LETTUCE   Emotional stillness; for issues preventing sleep and proper rest.

ORANGE   For hope; despair due to hormonal shifts; feeling overwhelmed by symptoms; inability to cope.

PEACH   "Poor me" attitude; for giving to others to the point of exhaustion; realizing that giving to yourself is equally as important; honoring the importance of caring for your special needs.

PEAR   "Emotional earthquakes"; feeling shaky, uncentered; for emergencies of any kind; sudden changes due to hormonal shifts.

PINEAPPLE	Self-trust to replace self doubt; for the ability to turn symptoms into tools for self-enhancement; self-image issues; for emotional reactions to weight gain.
RASPBERRY	For oversensitive feelings; remaining non-reactive to other people's shortcomings; sensitivity to other people's joys and pains.
SPINACH	To not take symptoms/changes too seriously; to make light of the many psycho-physical transformations.
STRAWBERRY	To understand your new role during and after menopause, to adjust with dignity to the new messages of your body and mind, also to resolve any lingering sell-worth issues triggered by menopause.
TOMATO	For stability while adjusting to different medications, to be strengthened and personally empowered by the opportunities for growth which menopause offers.

TREATING CODEPENDENCE WITH FLOWER ESSENCES

Now, to address another globally pervasive issue. Codependence is a new word for an old pattern that we would call a *dysfunction*. What does dysfunction mean? To be dysfunctional means to be disconnected from our feelings. We may, for example, fear abandonment in a relationship but, instead of recognizing that feeling and discussing it with the person with whom we are in a relationship, we might express anger instead. A functional person, on the other hand, would recognize and be in touch with a feeling, analyze what's behind it, and then be able to explain that feeling and its origins to another person.

Codependence, basically, is dysfunctional nurturing. Both men and women do it, though the typical male pattern is to withdraw and deny any needs altogether. Dysfunctional caregiving creates dependence; healthy nurturing encourages independence. The codependent individual typically comes from a dysfunctional home, that can usually be traced back through many generations. These familial symptoms include any or all of the following: alcohol or drug abuse; physical, emotional or sexual abuse; excessive arguing and resultant tension; and compulsive behaviors such as overworking, dieting, or gambling. All of these behaviors preclude honest intimacy.

Codependence is a form of addiction—not to substances but to other people, making it far more subtle and complex than many other addictions. For this reason, codependence requires longer to recover from than substance abuse. A codependent relationship may form between a mother and child, a friend and friend, with a lover, spouse or sibling, or even between a customer and car mechanic. Codependent individuals in very small or great ways tend to react, blame, feel powerless, depend on outside circumstances to make things right within themselves, deny and control, are denied and controlled, and basically seek answers and confirmation outside of their own inner wisdom. They are, in a word, emotionally infected with character weaknesses that lead head-long into suffering. The beauty of such lives go unclaimed, unacknowledged, and unexpressed.

This sounds serious and very "stuck." In order to apply the art of flower essences successfully, it's helpful to understand this explanation of the codependent personality. Emerging from codependence is a one-step-at-a-time process. Our history is not our destiny. We *can* reinvent ourselves. Let's remember the power we *do* have: the power to take charge of our lives, to be loving and whole. Beneath the superficial mud of dysfunction lies the perfect diamond of our true nature. The supportive message of flower essences is simple: *we can heal.* The following list offers some "essential" guidelines for help.

SPIRIT-IN-NATURE ESSENCES APPLIED TO CODEPENDENCE

ALMOND	To calm an addictive personality; to withdraw from a sense of need; for obsessive/compulsive behaviors.
APPLE	For a healthy self-image; for cleansing destructive emotions.
AVOCADO	For consciously remembering to use the tools for becoming "undependent"; to be aware when old patterns surface.
BANANA	For perspective on the nature of independence; for acting instead of reacting; realizing we deserve neither blame nor credit.

BLACKBERRY	To provide deeper insight into symptoms and solutions; for pure, constructive thinking.
CHERRY	For cheerfulness during setbacks; to counteract the downward pull of addictive personalities in one's home and work environment.
COCONUT	For stamina to persevere; for sticking with support groups and other supportive measures.
CORN	For fostering the belief that every day is a new opportunity to be whole and happy; to break the illusion of "being stuck."
DATE	For acceptance of others' faults; for nurturing directed toward yourself.
FIG	To learn to accept and honor your own feelings; to not be too hard on yourself for "blowing it."
GRAPE	For finding the source of love within yourself rather than expecting others to provide that fulfillment.
LETTUCE	For clear communication of thoughts and feelings; expressing yourself creatively; for "knowing that one knows."
ORANGE	For hope; despair; for giving up; for faith to find systems that work, books, friends, groups and therapists.
PEACH	To serve others out of wholeness and not neediness; to serve yourself when there is genuine need; to become a healthy caregiver.
PEAR	For trauma or crisis; for difficult or abusive relationships.
PINEAPPLE	For self-confidence, specifically for work-related issues; to "let your light shine."
RASPBERRY	For forgivenesss of all past hurts, recently and from many years past; to create compassionate new patterns of being and behavior.
SPINACH	To recapture a lost childhood; to deal more lightly with ongoing, difficult issues.
STRAWBERRY	For beauty; to dissolve the need for approval; to cleanse guilt and self-blame; for damaged sense of self by role models in childhood.
TOMATO	For finding the inner courage and strength to become the loving, functional person you have always longed to be; also for addictions; facing and overcoming fears.

The Lighter Side

We have now more thoroughly examined a physiologically as well as a psychologically-based condition—menopause and codependence. Through this study, we can see the play between character strengths and weaknesses—and that self-improvement is fully within our power. Menopause and codependence, in this light, are opportunities for profound growth.

When we view our lives impersonally, we see only images of light and dark. Our joys and pains are like mere shadows on a movie screen. Flower essences help us to turn obstacles into opportunities and to become vibrantly whole in the process.

CHAPTER THIRTY-THREE

The Joyful Art of Consultation

*"One word frees us from all the weight and pain of life;
that word is love."*
—Sophocles

PRACTITIONER AWARENESS QUIZ

This chapter addresses some of the more common issues on the subject of consultation. As in preparing the essences, the first thing to prepare is yourself. You might review the following check-list, or Practitioner Awareness Quiz. Keep it handy while working with friends, clients, or yourself.

Check a number from zero to five, zero meaning that the statement does not apply to you, and five indicating that you strongly agree.

Statement	0 1 2 3 4 5
1. I am well rested.	
2. I am well fed—neither hungry nor stuffed.	
3. I am comfortable with the room temperature—neither too hot nor too cold.	
4. I left my worries and concerns at the door.	
5. I have no pressing needs or distractions.	
6. My energy is strong and clear.	
7. I have no personal needs about how the client responds.	
8. I am a good listener.	
9. I have no personal investment in the outcome of this session.	
10. My consultation room invites a sense of comfort and trust.	
11. I am free of judgment.	
12. My client is assured of complete confidentiality.	

Now total the numbers of your responses. A minimum of thirty-nine points is acceptable for optimum benefits. Higher numbers can indicate a more sensitively rendered consultation.

THE ROOM

A peaceful, secure consultation room is very important. Perhaps you have gone for a therapy session and remember in detail the inviting warmth of the treatment room. You too will want to create a location free from distractions such as ringing phones or children popping in—a place that instills a sense of safety. Be sure to avoid any public or crowded places. You'll want the consultation environment to work with you, not against you. Out-of-doors can be workable too—a secluded patch of lawn, a flower garden, or a shady spot under an oak tree's branches.

If you have an office, you might consider plants, a small bubbly fountain, incense, candles, comfortable chairs, soothing posters or paintings on the walls, a box of tissues, and soft instrumental music. Ask your client about the music and incense as you begin the session.

THE CONSULTATION

The purpose of a consultation is, basically, to create a relationship between your client and the essences and also to inspire and to uplift. Essence selection involves the intuition, which is like a muscle—the more you use it, the more it will develop. Practitioners employ many tools to access their intuition, including kinesiology (muscle testing) and dowsing. Or, you might simply try seeing yourself as a translator versed in the language of the flowers. Listen to your client ask in his own words, at least three times, for each essence.

"I'm not comfortable at home, even with all the doors safely locked. I'm still healing from past physical abuse. My nervous system feels wired for disaster." These three client statements point to the need for Pear, to help her feel "at home" within herself. Here's a helpful tip—if you are unable to "hear" your client ask for specific essences, Pear is a good first essence. It can initiate a clearing of consciousness and sensitize your client to the other essences in the program.

A SAMPLE CONSULTATION

You might try offering a program of five or six essences in a session, to be taken consecutively rather than concurrently, over the course of about four to six weeks. How to assess the length of time on each essence? Use the intuitive method that works best for you. I like to suggest to my clients, as a means of empowering and involving them, that five days, for example, means give or take two on either side, at their discretion. At the end of the program, the client may: (a) choose a follow-up session; (b) absorb and integrate the first program before beginning another; or (c) feel confident enough to work out his own self-assessed program and venture boldly into new essence waters, so to speak.

The theme essence usually falls last in the program and is generally taken for two weeks. This sequence allows the individual to peel back layers of issues before "coming home" to his theme essence. However, this is merely a suggested "essence road map." You may want to experiment with this method and then evolve your own style. To give an idea of the course a session may take, here is a humorous, fictionalized consultation with someone we all know, using the terms we have studied in the course of this book. Condensed into a short newspaper clipping, it might read as follows:

"Little Red Riding Hood takes a basket of goodies to her ailing grandmother. She is waylaid en route by a charming and urbane wolf. Wolf eats grandmother whole. Wolf disguises himself in grandmother's dressing gown and eats girl for dessert. Huntsman rescues girl and elder relative from wolf's belly, slings pelt across shoulders, and ambles home."

Were Little Red Riding Hood to schedule an appointment for a flower essence consultation, we might profile her case in the following way:

Little Red sauntered into my office this morning. A bouquet of wildflowers (that she had stopped to pick, thus making her ten minutes late for our appointment) burst from the famous basket she used to transport Grandma's goodies. She appeared a bit distracted and also distraught from the recent, and understandable, trauma that day. Her wide, trusting eyes flickered with a passing hint of suspicion. I observed her hesitation. She seemed out-of-sorts with herself—uncomfortable, as though she expected her aggressor to reappear momentarily.

Little Red retold the tale of her visit to Grandmother's in graphic detail—her mother's admonition not to dawdle or talk to strangers; the lovely scent of the sweetcakes and wine wafting up from the basket, matched by the windblown aroma of wildflowers along the forest trail; her kindliness in wanting to believe the wolf's foolery; not trusting her instincts to see her "grandmother" so visibly changed, i.e., "What big ears you have"; and the final blow of being devoured whole.

We then mapped out her essence program. Little Red initially required symptom treatment to deal with the series of events that had thrown her off balance. The first essence in her program was Pear for four days, to deal with the obvious shock and trauma of a fairly disastrous experience. Pear, as a peripheral plot essence, could help clear these disturbing cellular memories so that she needn't be frightened of other wolves in the future. (Remember, too, that Pear is an excellent first essence to prepare your client for the remainder of his program.) Tomato for five days, being a second peripheral plot essence, would reinforce Pear's initial clearing. Addressing any residual fear, Tomato could help Little Red to bounce back more completely. "Undefeated in every trial" is Tomato's message.

We added one further peripheral plot essence—Blackberry, for one week. Purification being its key quality, this essence could help her to view the recent trauma as a mere bad dream with no lingering effects to her psyche.

Then we arrived at a turning point in her essence program. Little Red was now ready to move to a core treatment approach and to deal with more longstanding life issues. Forgetting her mother's warning not to wander off or speak to strangers; losing her sense of direction and purpose in the forest; distracted by wildflowers: three times over, she is asking for her pivotal plot essence, Avocado, to be taken for one week and repeated at a later date, as pivotal plot indications recur throughout our lives. Little Red shared during the course of our visit that she routinely lost her homework assignments or turned them in incomplete because they were not challenging enough. Her mother called her absent-minded, indicating a pivotal Avocado plot essence.

Little Red's Raspberry theme essence concluded our first program, recommended for two weeks, also to be repeated in the future, much like her pivotal plot essence. She was not only kind and loving to her grandmother, which initiated her trip through the woods in the first place, but was loved by all who knew her as kindhearted and considerate to playmates and woodland animal friends alike. Raspberry themes see kindness everywhere. Thus she even saw a kindliness in the wicked wolf. A note of interest—the raspberry-colored cloak that she wears every day is another clue to her theme essence.

If she should desire a follow-up consultation, Spinach would undoubtedly be useful to restore her trust and balance it with common sense; to reinforce her childhood innocence; and finally, to ensure an unscarred early life so that she might grow to functional, healthy adulthood and beyond.

As for the wolf—had he survived his own treachery, we would have employed core treatment with a focus on Raspberry as his pivotal plot essence, for the ultimate unkindness of eating people whole; suggested Grape as a peripheral plot essence to counteract his ruthlessness and cunning; and offered Blackberry, another peripheral plot essence, to help him counteract his deception of both Little Red and her unsuspecting grandmother.

A WELL-ORCHESTRATED CONSULTATION

To summarize, here are eight keys to a well-presented session. I have added essences to thematically illustrate these points. You may wish to include other elements that you find especially helpful.

Safety—Tomato: An environment that is comforting and comfortable says more than words —that here is a place to let your guard down, to heal, and to regain inner strength.

Trust—Spinach: The sensitive practitioner creates a place where each client feels comfortable and relaxed and that who he is, is okay. The healing process is a shared adventure.

Confidentiality—Strawberry: Without respect for the client's privacy, no progress is possible. This warrants a high level of integrity on the practitioner's part.

Acceptance—Date: There should be no judgment or blame in your office, either toward the client or those of whom he speaks.

Listening—Banana: Many, many times, this is what people need most. To be heard is a vital part of your client's healing process.

Support—Apple: To present a more holistic program, offer the corresponding *Essence Enhancers, Visualizations,* and *Affirmations,* and the Spirit-in-Nature *Essence Songs* CD.

Inspiration—Coconut: Remember, we may have faults, but we are not our shortcomings. Inspire your client with a sense of his highest potential and innate inner wellbeing.

Hope—Orange: There is always hope, always light at the end of the darkest tunnel. Joy is our true nature. Be sure this message is conveyed to your client, both verbally and vibrationally!

Following this chapter, you will find several pages—a consultation form, the client's copy of the essence program, and a flower essences response sheet. Feel free to duplicate them with the copyright.

Theme Essence_____ Name_____

Theme Essence Food _____

Date_____ Address _____

City/State/Zip_____ Phone _____

Birth Date_____ Marital Status_____ Children _____

Initial Consultation ☐ Phone ☐ In Person ☐ Letter

Previous PE Experience_____ No _____

Occupation _____

1. Essence_____ Duration _____

_____

2. Essence_____ Duration _____

_____

3. Essence_____ Duration _____

_____

4. Essence_____ Duration _____

_____

5. Essence_____ Duration _____

_____

Physical Health (include history of illness/accident/surgery) _____

_____

_____

Emotional Health (include history of childhood issues/trauma) _____

_____

_____

Relationship Issues (past/present) _____

_____

Notes _____

_____

_____

_____

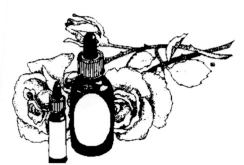

Roadmap to
Inner Well-being

Program #:_____ Theme Essence_____ Date_____

      Theme Essence: Plot Essence: Duration:

1. _____ _____ _____

Notes: _____

_____

      Theme Essence: Plot Essence: Duration:

2. _____ _____ _____

Notes: _____

_____

      Theme Essence: Plot Essence: Duration:

3. _____ _____ _____

Notes: _____

_____

      Theme Essence: Plot Essence: Duration:

4. _____ _____ _____

Notes: _____

      Theme Essence: Plot Essence: Duration:

5. _____ _____ _____

Notes: _____

_____

14618 Tyler Foote Road   •   Nevada City, CA 95959 USA   •   Phone 530.478.7655

Spirit-in-Nature Essences

For Perfect Well-being

Spirit-in-Nature Essences Response Sheet

This evaluation form will be used to gather research information on Spirit-in-Nature Essences. At your request, it will be held in strict confidence. When you notice specific results from your program, please complete this form and return it to: Spirit-in-Nature Essences, 14618 Tyler Foote Road, Nevada City, CA 95959. *(Questions? Call us at: 530.478.7655.)* Feel free to write on another sheet of paper if necessary. Thank you for your reply that will help us compile future literature.

THIS SECTION OPTIONAL:

Name _____

Date_____ Phone ( ) _____

Address _____

City _____ State _____ Zip_____

Birthdate_____ Marital status _____ ____ Ages of children_____

Why do you feel drawn to using *Spirit-in-Nature Essences?* I am taking these *(list specific name)* essences: _____

☐ to develop the particular quality that it addresses

☐ because I am already strong in that quality and want to develop it even further

☐ to help me with a certain issue/test

☐ as a preventive healing

☐ to assist in a major life change

☐ for a physical health-related issue

☐ for clarifying mental/emotional issues

☐ for enhancing my personal growth

☐ for emergency use

☐ other

Please explain your choice(s) listed above: _____

_____

_____

_____

14618 Tyler Foote Road • Nevada City, CA 95959 USA • Phone 530.478.7655

How often do/did you take *Spirit-in-Nature Essences?*_____times daily

Please list exact times of the day: _____ _____

Dates taken: From: _____ to _____

Please describe your results in detail *(when you first experienced them, how you were affected)*.

_____

_____

_____

_____

State your reasons for attributing these results to *Spirit-in-Nature Essences* and not to other

causes:_____

_____

_____

_____

Are you presently using other forms of treatment/supplements? *(please list).* _____

_____

_____

_____

Please explain any significant events/changes/outlooks in your life that prompted you to take

Spirit-in-Nature Essences: _____

_____

_____

_____

How you selected your *Spirit-in-Nature Essence(s):*
☐ Flower Essence practitioner *(please list method of diagnosis)*
☐ Consultation: ? other:
☐ muscle testing *(kinesiology)*
☐ radiesthesia *(dowsing)*
☐ intuitive selection
☐ study of *Spirit-in-Nature Essences*
☐ other *(please list):*
☐ Please keep the above information in strict confidence
☐ You may use the above evaluation
☐ with my name;
☐ anonymously, for testimonials and upcoming literature

Signature_____ Date_____

CHAPTER THIRTY-FOUR

LITTLE BLOSSOMS: OUR CHILDREN

"A simple child,
That lightly draws its breath,
And feels life in every limb,
What should it know of death?" —Wordsworth

AN ENERGETIC BRIDGE

There is a cartoon of a father teaching his son to ride a bicycle. The father asks his son, who is understandably shaky on the bike, to trust him. "Trust you?" the boy asks. "I've only known you six years!" It's this charming simplicity that allows children to respond so quickly to flower essences. Even lifelong patterns can be changed with a single dosage. When we as adults in the role of caregivers are aware of our children's realities—their needs, their joys, and their pains—then we can effectively minister to them through Nature's delicate gift of flower essences to nuture them as "little blossoms."

Developmentally, children pass through four stages that usher them to the doorstep of adulthood. Each of these stages presents different challenges to the child. From birth to age seven, children learn about the physical world through their bodies and their senses. From age seven to twelve, roughly, they are developing their feeling and emotional nature and beginning to understand the world on subtler levels. From age twelve to eighteen, they deal with power and the raw will of adolescence as they begin their search for self-identity. From eighteen to twenty-four, they focus more on developing the reasoning side of their nature.

Flower essences are effective catalysts for children to grow more fully in each important developmental stage. They are also an excellent way for us, as adults, to get in touch with any hidden agendas within our own inner child that have not been healed. For this reason it is a good idea for parents and children to take essences together, oftentimes the same ones. Here, we would look at the needs of the household as a single entity as well as at the component parts of the individuals who comprise it.

So often children, especially younger ones, will act out and mirror their parents' difficulties. Sharing essences helps to create an energetic bridge between parent and child, bringing clarity to each person individually as well as to the relationships between family members. Peach, for example, is helpful for older children when a new sibling arrives. It can help them to feel emotionally secure in the changing climate of an expanding family.

Dosage directions for children are the same as for adults. Administer their dosage in juice, water, or baby's bottle. You may find your kids asking for their essences and making sure you remember to dispense them!

LITTLE BLOSSOM THEMES

Although it may seem more difficult to decipher a child's theme essence than an adult's, it can actually be easier. Children live their strengths, and thus their themes, candidly and conspicuously. Food cravings are an excellent clue as well. The Peach theme child, for example, shares her dolls at an early age—or even gives them away to other children less fortunate. The Grape theme child excels in the art of hugging. And the Avocado theme hardly seems a child at all, being more of the wise old man or the tribal crone, even from birth!

Caroline, a five-year-old Orange theme, speaks freely about herself:

"If my friends aren't happy, I do something funny. If I wasn't happy, I would go swing on the swingset, or I'd look at the rainbows on the wall. I smile a lot because I'm happy. I'm happy because I'm a Sagittarius. And going skiing with my dad makes me happy. I'm *not* happy when it rains because I don't want to have to wear a raincoat when I have a ponytail in my hair. I like it when snow comes 'cause I like my comfy snowsuit.

"Oranges are juicy. I hold them up to my mouth. I like oranges and orange juice. I didn't eat oranges when I was a teensy-tinesy baby. I never drank out of a bottle. I never ate until I was talking."

Caroline's mother speaks:

"Well, she's very joyful. She's a very happy child. She always has been, ever since birth. She just smiled a lot and loved everybody and everything. She's like a little pixie, a little sprite. If she's afraid of something or someone, then she might cry. Or if she's got low blood sugar or is tired, then she'll cry. She knows it's okay to cry but that it's also okay for her to try and change her energy. To do that, she goes and secludes for a little bit in her room. 'Uh uh,' Caroline interjects. 'I get a drink of water. Sometimes when you tell me to go to my room, I sneak out and get a drink.' And then she comes back cheerful and loving."

Some years ago, a mother of two children shared a rather unusual story about her daughter, a Raspberry theme:

"From the time I was two months pregnant until I was literally wheeled into the delivery room, I craved raspberries—that have never before or since been especially important to me. I bought anything at the grocery with raspberries in it, including fresh ones out of season at five dollars a basket! I would make raspberry sauce for baked chicken, eat raspberry yogurt, raspberry popsicles—anything!

"Well, my daughter, Kasey, who's five now, is about the kindest child you could imagine. She spends an hour at a time caring for her 'little babies,' telling me, 'Oh, Mama, they're too hot,' or 'Mama, they're too cold!' And she *loves* raspberries. Her bedroom is painted a deep pink. She dresses herself in pink, and she has the same craving for raspberries that I did when I was pregnant!"

LITTLE BLOSSOM PLOTS

Plot essences are fairly transparent for children. Just watch kids manifest their needs without veil or pretense! Peripheral plot essence issues surface quickly in the form of accidents, trouble at school and the inevitable conflicts with siblings and friends. And pivotal plots, like their theme counterparts, make themselves known through behavior patterns from a very early age.

Peripheral plot essences surface regularly and often for children. "We use Pineapple for soccer games," says the mother of eight-year-old Alan. "I also put Pineapple in the drinking water on our river rafting trip. It has 'I think I can' energy in it. On the trip, Alan said, 'Gimme that!' He loves it."

Carlen is an Avocado theme with Peach as his pivotal plot essence. In his own words, here's why:

"I love drawing. I've been drawing for, like, all my life. I'm ten now. It's fun, you can draw anything you want. I sort of look around the room and see what I want to draw. Like a telephone might look like an army machine or a space cadet because of the antenna. I like drawing plants. They have lots of details. There's a lot of shading, I like shading.

"My favorite subject at school is computer class. I like typing stories into the computer. I have a good memory. I remember phone numbers if I see them once or twice. I had a test about my memory. You look at this picture with about twenty things you have to remember, and then there are fifteen questions on the next page. I only got one wrong.

"I daydream sometimes. Like, if my mom said, 'go make the bed,' I might lie down and read a book because I forgot about it. Also, I'd like to have some friends that I like a little better that would just come over."

Carlen's pivotal plot, Peach, expresses itself through his need (quite common in most children!) to be more sensitive to his mother. With Peach clearing his magnetism to include the sensitivities of others, he could then draw the friends he seeks. Fortunately, Carlen's father is a Peach sub-theme and their bond proves very strengthening for him.

INTERPRETATIONS FOR CHILDREN

The following list offers some guidelines for essence application for our "little blossoms." Read through the following list and feel free to add your own experiential definitions.

ALMOND—Self-control, including control of sexual energies; for peer pressure; calmness; beneficial to preteens while establishing their identities as they mature into adulthood.

APPLE—Clarity; healthfulness; may be administered during illness or when the thought of illness is present; for periods of discouragement.

AVOCADO—Good memory; for the child who forgets his chores, his manners, or his personal habits; helps with school work; sharpens concentration; for learning musical instruments or undertaking creative endeavors.

BANANA—Humility; calmness; for the child who needs to center his attention less on himself and more on family and friends.

BLACKBERRY—Purity of thought; for the "terrible two's"; and for children who have been exposed to harmful movies, games, or television programs; for more positive, wholesome thoughts.

CHERRY—Cheerfulness; for the child prone to moods or periods of withdrawal; for times of sadness or disappointment; helps heal the trauma of divorce, imminent or past; for bed-wetting.

COCONUT—Uplifted spiritual awareness; helps a child deal with sibling rivalry; for times of challenge or struggle in school or in group dynamics; for maturity and the ability to make better choices in life, especially in difficult situations.

CORN—Mental vitality; for new beginnings: a new school year, moving to a new location, making new friends; for encouragement and a burst of energy; for "the study blahs'"; for carsickness.

DATE—Sweetness, tenderness; for the child with a sour disposition who is overly critical or judgmental of others; for the child who finds fault with others (siblings especially); for whining, clinging children.

FIG—Flexibility; self-acceptance; for the child who is too hard on him- self or tries too hard; for being unsatisfied with accomplishments even when they are noteworthy; for the ability to see many sides of an issue; for nail-biting and thumb-sucking.

GRAPE—Love; a remedy for any attitude that is not loving; for the bully or the tattletale; for tantrums.

LETTUCE—Calmness; for children who don't like salad; helps children when they are too "wound up" to play constructively; for sleeplessness; the essence to take before oral exams and recitals.

ORANGE—enthusiasm; for hope; to help dispels deep moods; discontentment; helpful during teething; for emotional issues connected with any accidents to the head; promotes an active interest in life.

PEACH—Unselfishness; concern for the welfare of others; excellent for the weaning process; promotes a sense of sharing and cooperation with other children.

PEAR—Emergency essence; for accidents, sudden illness, or any crisis situation; helps with toilet training; facilitates the learning of positive new habits; for children who have a hard time listening in school or to their parents; for fidgety, restless energy.

PINEAPPLE—Self-assurance; helps to "untie the apron strings"; for the child who has been singled out by peers for being smaller, larger, or in some way different; for the child who is painfully shy.

RASPBERRY—Kindness; compassion; for the child who hurts others or is easily hurt; for over-sensitivity; promotes a giving nature.

SPINACH—Simplicity; for the child who is prematurely grown up or overly-serious; for times of stress, exhaustion or overwork; for those situations in which a child feels distraught or overwhelmed.

STRAWBERRY—Dignity; for the child who has trouble letting go of being a baby; for a deep sense of self-worth; helps with clarity of self-image; for the child dealing with divorce of parents.

TOMATO—Mental strength, courage; endurance; helps to dissolve fears; for children who suffer from nightmares; helps children to move forward in their lives when they are anxious, nervous, or unwilling.

IN CONCLUSION

There is so much more to say on the subject of children and flower essences that my hope someday is to devote an entire book to essences for families. These little blossoms, entrusted to our care, are a sacred part of our own life journey. Children are our present and our priceless future. George Bernard Shaw worded it well: "Perhaps the greatest service that can be rendered by anybody to the country and to mankind, is to bring up a family."

CHAPTER THIRTY-FIVE

Four-Footed Friends
and Other Critters:
Pets and Animals

"Arise from sleep, old cat,
And with great yawns and stretchings—
Amble out for love." —Kobayashi Issa

"A small bird flew into my house and, because of the open look of sliding glass doors, crashed into it, stunning himself badly. I gave him spring water with Pear and in fifteen minutes he was on the wing again. One other almost identical circumstance occurred with another bird of a much larger species. The bird was in *severe* shock. After several drops of Pear, he came to consciousness again and regained his balance. After twenty minutes, he was airborne." —*MLB, La Honda, CA*

"My fourteen-year-old cat, Jasmine, had been traumatized and ripped up by a dog. I think it made her nasty. She's absolutely sweet when she drinks her water with Grape added to it, and started going outside for the first time in two years. The Grape keeps her loving."
—*SR, Santa Clara, CA*

"In May, my Arabian mare birthed her new foal in a pasture in the dark on a cold and windy evening. I was awakened by her frantic neighing. Her new son, trying out his wobbly legs, had rolled under the fence and into the adjacent pasture. Instantly I had them both on Pear to calm them, and calm them it did." —*RR, Reno, Nevada*

"My six-year-old cat, Rusty, was abandoned as a kitten and doesn't know how to handle love. He also has a nervous skin condition. With Lettuce in his water, he drinks twice as much, and after only three or four days, is much more calm and less needy."   —LC, Richmond, VA

RABBITS TO ROADRUNNERS

How readily animals have crept into our language. We "chicken out," "horse around," or "pig out" and then act catty or sheepish until someone "gets our goat." Cartoons and caricatures have long drawn on the humor of attributing human qualities to animals and vice versa. We might remember the hippos in tutus, the super hero Mighty Mouse, or the numerous talking pigs, rabbits, and roadrunners who inundated the cinematic screens of our childhood.

The animal kingdom, so intricately linked to the plant kingdom, holds a special place in this world. From predators to friends, animals are a part of our lives. We see them in zoos, on leashes, in captivity, and in the wilds. Animals, like flowers and people, are living blossoms possessed of life force with their own special secrets to share with us. A young East Indian woman saint, Bahina, said of her pet cow that she could "understand every action of the calf as a child understands the language of its pet. If you have love enough to understand, you can interpret every movement of the animals."[15] Here Bahina echoes the universal truth expressed by George Washington Carver that anything will give up its secrets if you love it enough. And what treasures we can learn from our animal friends!

Pets—domesticated animals who are our companions—open our hearts and expand our consciousness. Much like one direct experience with a flower essence can open the entire essence world for us, so too a deep connection with even one animal allows us to access the spirit of their kingdom. One of the dearest times of my life was spent as a back-to-the-land goat herder. To this day, I remain grateful to the goats who befriended me several decades ago. They have enriched my life, my appreciation for Nature, and my ability to love, immeasurably. Like a direct hot line to nature's simple rhythms, the melodic act of milking put me in touch with the pulse of the animal kingdom.

Interestingly, it was not until Jane Goodall's pioneering work with chimpanzees in the early sixties that the scientific world acknowledged what pet owners have known all along—that animals experience a wide range of feelings. These include joy, hope, grief, and—as observed in bears sitting on their haunches meditatively absorbed in a sunset panorama—an appreciation of beauty. The joy of performing dolphins who *ad lib* on their own acts; the grievous weeping of a circus elephant after being punished for not responding; the goose who gestures and articulates victory, uncertainty, tension, and alertness: who are we to call animals dumb? Their wisdom is an intuition born of instinct, a sort of intact umbilical cord to Mother Nature.

It is this wealth of an emotional repertoire that allows animals to respond so beautifully to their "flower friends" in essence form. Granted, consultation as we know it is not possible with animals. But those who are sensitive know that animals communicate with us constantly through their sounds, gestures, postures, and actions. Like children, animals whom we have domesticated are dependent on us for their psycho-physical well-being. Flower essence interpretations in the children's chapter may be applied to them as well. And as with children and parents, pets and their owners may either need to share the same essences or be on essence programs at the same time. Let's not underestimate the instinctual intuition of our animal friends, who sense our nervousness and our joy alike, oftentimes before we ourselves do. One woman recently called for essences for her six-year-old dog who had been bitten by a rattlesnake a year ago. Rascal had been suffering from *grand mal* seizures ever since. We talked about a program for him and Pear, immediately, for her!

The death of a beloved pet is a subject in itself. Flower essences can assist both the animal and the family, who must go through their grieving and adjust to life without their dear companion. Bonnie, teary-eyed, shared this story only a few days ago:

"Yesterday, our nine-year-old cat had to be put to sleep. Calicos are known for being the wildest of the cat family. Our kitty had apparently climbed up on the roof, fallen, and broken her back. The vet called in tears to say he had just put her to sleep moments before our teenage daughter arrived. She'd gone into uncontrollable spasms and seizures. Needless to say, we were badly shaken. My whole family, plus the cat up until her passing, have been on Pear. I can't tell you how much it has helped. It allowed us to stay centered and deal with this trauma in a peaceful way." (Note: after the immediate shock of a pet's passing clears, Grape is an excellent follow-up essence.)

Practical Application

Follow the directions of four Stock drops daily in a cup of water and sixteen drops to a water tub for horses and large animals. In emergency situations, you can apply the essence topically on the coat, fur, feathers, or scales. It's not necessary to force the drops into their mouths and it may be difficult to isolate their water supply from their food dish. Not to worry. Since animals respond to essences even more rapidly than children, dropping the essences into their water bowl works fine. You might also spray their coats and bedding—four Stock drops to a misting bottle—or gently rub essences on bruised or sprained areas.

Like Father, Like Son

Animals who spend time around humans begin to develop their own personalities. Many cartoons have played off the theme of how much dog owners resemble their dogs—sometimes psychologically, sometimes in fact, physically. Much like children, pets mirror their masters' strengths and weaknesses. A standoffish owner, for instance, can foster an aloof animal; a demonstrative one is reflected in an overly-affectionate or clingy pet. For this reason, you might treat the owner along with the pet! I have talked with many a vet who has traced his patients' problems directly back to their owners.

In addition to individual differences, the various species express a variety of mass consciousness characteristics. Cats share a certain aloofness that British comedic writer P. G. Wodehouse attributes to their not having gotten over being deified in ancient Egypt. Dogs, as a rule, have earned the title of "man's best friend." Cows are ruminatively slow and goats are endlessly capricious. It is helpful to take into account these species similarities when administering flower essences to animals. With animals as well as humans, we want to nurture their existing strengths and not try to make them over into something they were never instinctively wired to be. Remember, flower essences will *enhance* an animal's innate personality; they will not manipulate or control it.

With a little sensitivity, we can detect when a cat needs Coconut, to adjust to the arrival of new cats in the household or Grape, when the older hamster bullies the younger one. Grape is also helpful for the pet who whines from loneliness—although whining from being a bit spoiled indicates Peach! Pear is very popular for accidents or injuries, as well as for transporting animals from one location to another in a vehicle that is foreign to them, or for pets who simply don't travel well. Tomato works wonderfully for the cat who has been moved to a new home, an experience that can be severely disorienting for her. To determine the essence needs of animals, you might try the pendulum, kinesiology, or simply "listening" with your heart. So too, our every kindness—through gentle words, a loving touch, and the sensitive use of flower essences—hastens them on their spiritual journey toward greater freedom.

CHAPTER THIRTY-SIX

FINDING THE ESSENCE OF LIFE

"The black squares on a checkerboard alternate with the white. Even so, every darkness in life alternates with light, every sorrow with a joy, every failure with a success. Change and contrast are inevitable, and are what make the great game possible. View them dispassionately, and never allow them to define who you are, inwardly." —Paramhansa Yogananda

THE GREAT GAME

"You have to live anyway," Yogananda said. "Why not live in the right way?" Each of the following guidelines for right living paraphrases one of the Spirit-in-Nature Essences.

LETTUCE: Be calm. Let your thoughts, words and actions flow from a quiescent place within you. Let your presence be calming to others.

COCONUT: Know that inherent in every problem is its solution. The answers you seek to life's challenges lie within your ability to perceive the questions. Live an inspired and inspirational life.

CHERRY: Be happy! Resolve in your mind that no one and nothing can rob you of this happiness.

SPINACH: Let the child within you come out and play. Skip, dance, or sing. Above all, don't take yourself or anyone else too seriously.

PEACH: Be sensitive to the needs of others. Give from your own inner wholeness; love for the sake of loving.

CORN: Put energy into *everything* you do; energy begets energy. Affirm that you have more than enough vitality to accomplish any task set before you.

TOMATO: Make it a habit to act from your strengths. Empower yourself with the thought that you are bigger than any trial and thus victorious.

PINEAPPLE: Know yourself, and know that you know. Life is your friend; greet it as such with straightforward confidence.

BANANA: Be little in your greatness and goodness. Always be willing to step out of the way and view yourself as a mere passing event for which you are responsible.

FIG: Roll with the punches. Be flexible in your habits and attitudes. Be not self-limiting, but rather self-liberating. You may have to live with yourself a long time, so enjoy your own company!

ALMOND: Interiorize your mind. Be the master of your senses and desires instead of vice versa. Commit your energy with great vigor in every endeavor.

PEAR: Choose to remain unruffled, even in the most extenuating circumstances. Become the cure instead of the malady.

AVOCADO: Wake up! Be interested in your life, the lives of others, and in life itself. Never stop learning, questioning, or creating.

APPLE: Bring the crispness of an apple to your thoughts. Fill your mind with a diet of positive, life-affirming attitudes. Do a cleansing fast from all worries.

ORANGE: "Smile, and the world smiles with you." Forget everything that has made you unhappy. Smile until it hurts.

BLACKBERRY: Hold the image of yourself as taintless, like a crystal clear window. Instead of reflecting off of you, imagine light radiating out from within and through you. Identify with that light.

DATE: Resolve to see everything around you as sweet. Reach out to people, and allow yourself to be touched in return. Judge no one; accept everyone just as they are. What we see is what we become.

STRAWBERRY: Hold your body with poise. Speak from quiet integrity. Realize that whatever has happened to you in the past, good or bad, has no bearing on the present. Know that, as you are respectful of others, you are also deserving of their respect.

RASPBERRY: Forgive your transgressors. Forgive yourself. Act from wholeness instead of reacting from woundedness. Above all, live kindly.

 GRAPE: Be loving, and you will be supremely lovable. Let love be the depth and breadth of your existence.

THE BEGINNING

Flower essences are at our disposal, ultimately, to remind us of our innate perfection. In gentle, non-invasive ways, they tell us that we already *are* our highest potential. We need only to realize this truth.

In the words of Thoreau, "Every man is his own masterpiece." May these essences serve you well as tools with which to sculpt your life and assist you in your service to others. Truly, life is a checkerboard, resplendent with alternating segments of light and dark, poverty and prosperity, health and sickness, sorrow and joy. With equanimity, poise and balance, we come to understand our part in it all.

CHAPTER THIRTY-SEVEN

RECIPES

JUST FOR FUN

"Restore me with raisins, comfort me with apples; for I am sick with love." —Old Testament, Song of Solomon

You will find these recipes in harmony with the nature of flower essences— surprisingly delightful and uncommonly simple. Perhaps you'll want to explore them along with their corresponding essences.

Almond Pudding

1 c. almonds, blanched in boiling water

1 qt. milk

1 pt. cream

2-3 T. semolina flour, or cream of wheat

1/2 c. turbinado sugar or 1/3 c. honey

1 t. almond extract

Soak almonds overnight. Remove skins by rubbing with a rough, clean dish towel. Blend almonds with milk until very smooth. Strain. Add cream and cook in a heavy pot over medium heat until boiling. Add semolina flour and sugar, boiling gently until reduced by 1/3. Add almond extract. Cool.

Baked Apples

6 apples
1/2 c. chopped walnuts
1/2 c. raisins
1 T. cinnamon
1/2 c. honey

Choose tart baking apples such as pippins, one per person. Wash and core. In a small bowl mix walnuts, raisins, cinnamon, and honey. Stuff apples with mixture and bake on a buttered baking dish for 35 to 40 minutes.

Avocado Dressing

1 ripe avocado
1/2 lemon, juiced
1 c. water
1 clove fresh garlic
t. whole coriander seeds
t. olive oil

Blend and serve over your favorite greens.

Spiced Bananas

There are many varieties of bananas—some with hints of other fruit flavors. Plantains are one type you might find in American grocery stores. Try them, or the more traditional variety, for this recipe.

2 T. butter or ghee
1/4 t. nutmeg, freshly ground if possible
1/2 t. cinnamon
1/2 t. cardamon
1/2 c. raisins or currants
4 bananas cut into rounds or strips
Hot whole grain cereal
Vanilla ice cream

Heat butter or ghee in heavy skillet on low heat. Add spices and raisins and cook for 5 minutes, until the raisins plump up and absorb the spices. Add the bananas and stir, cooking for 1 minute more. Spoon over cereal or ice cream.

Blackberry Pie

Pie crust (compliments of *Simply Vegetarian*):

3/4 c. whole wheat pastry flour

3/4 c. unbleached white flour 1 cube cold butter

Preheat oven to 325 degrees. Mix the above ingredients in large bowl with a pastry cutter or two knives.

Slowly add 3 T. cold water, tossing mixture with a fork to distribute water evenly, until the mixture holds together. Cut in half. Roll out half of mixture on a lightly floured board. Place in 9″ pie pan.

Filling:

4-5 c. fresh or 1 qt. canned blackberries

c. turbinado sugar or 2/3 c. honey

T. cornstarch (3 T. if honey is used) dissolved in 1/2 c. cold water

cinnamon to taste

Mix together the above ingredients. Pour into unbaked crust. Sprinkle with cinnamon. Use second crust to make lattice topping. Flute the edges. Bake for 30 to 40 minutes at 325 degrees.

Cherry Sauce

This will cheer up just about anything! Pour over poundcake, ice cream or fruit salad.

2 lbs. fresh dark sweet cherries

1 c. cherry cider or juice

t. lemon juice

dash cinnamon

t. cornstarch, dissolved in 1/2 c. cold water

Pit cherries and set aside. Bring juice to boil, add lemon, cinnamon, and honey. Add dissolved cornstarch, stirring with wire whisk. When thick, remove from heat, add cherries, and serve.

Coconut Rice

For dessert or breakfast!

1 c. coconut milk (canned) OR make by blending 1/2 c. dried coconut with 1 c. boiling water

1 c. basmati rice

1 c. water

Wash rice, place with water and coconut milk in a saucepan, and bring to a boil. Turn heat down to lowest setting and simmer, covered, for 20 minutes until all the liquid is absorbed. Garnish with toasted coconut.

Roasted Corn

Remove the corn silk, leaving the husks on the corn. Soak them in water for 10 minutes. Tie them shut with a twist-tie. Place them over hot coals on a barbecue, turning them after 5 minutes. Open and squeeze the juice of 1/4 lime on each ear of corn. If you like, sprinkle on some cayenne. (This is a traditional Caribbean recipe.)

Stuffed Dates

20 whole dates

1/2 c. cream cheese

20 walnut or pecan halves

1/2 c. coconut

Choose moist, whole dates. Slice open to remove pits but keep whole. Fill inside with cream cheese and top with a walnut half. Roll in coconut and serve.

Fresh Figs with Dip

20 fresh figs

1/2 c. ricotta cheese

1 t. honey

1 t. cardamon

4-6 fresh mint leaves

Arrange figs on a platter. Stir honey and cardamon into ricotta cheese Garnish with mint leaves. Use as a dip for fresh figs.

Frozen Grapes

This is one of the easiest possible recipes—so add lots of love!

Wash grapes and pop them into the freezer for one hour. Be sure to use seedless grapes. These are great for car trips on hot summer days. Enjoy!

Spring Rolls Wrapped in Lettuce

Wrapping freshly cooked spring rolls in lettuce is a delight to the palate.

Shredded fresh lettuce, cabbage, and carrots

Finely chopped celery

1 T. oil

1 T. fresh ginger

1 qt. peanut oil

Egg roll wrappers

Lettuce leaves

Sweet and sour sauce

Quickly stir-fry veggies in 1 T. oil with fresh ginger. Wrap in egg roll wrappers and fry in peanut oil until golden brown. Wrap each in a lettuce leaf and serve with sweet and sour sauce.

Orange Salad

2 blood oranges

c. jicama chunks

c. fresh baby greens

2 T. olive oil

1 T. balsamic vinegar

Mix together and serve well chilled.

Peach Cobbler

Filling:

6-8 fresh peaches peeled and sliced into glass baking dish

1/2 c. honey, poured evenly over peaches

Topping:

c. butter

c. flour

1 c. granola

1/2 c. chopped almonds

Mix together and sprinkle on top of filling. Bake one hour at 325 degrees.

Gingered Pears

4-6 ripe fresh pears

1 t. grated fresh ginger

1/2 c. honey

Vanilla ice cream

Slice and peel pears, arranging in a fan shape in a glass baking dish. Sprinkle with ginger and drizzle honey over the top. Bake for 20 minutes at 300 degrees.

Serve with vanilla ice cream.

Pineapple Fluff

fresh pineapple, cored, and finely chopped

c. cooked millet, cooled

1 pt. whipped cream

1 t. cardamon powder

Mix together and chill well. This makes a great breakfast or dessert.

Raspberry Butter

2 c. raspberries (1 basket)

1/2 c. unsalted butter

Wash raspberries. Run through a fine mesh sieve to remove seeds. Soften 1/2 c. butter to room temperature. Next add raspberry sauce to butter, mixing well. Serve with bagels, on French toast, or waffles.

Cream of Spinach Soup

bunch fresh spinach

qts. soup stock

1 carrot, diced

1 celery stalk, chopped finely

1 small onion, diced

1 stick cinnamon

4 cloves

1 T. fresh ginger

1 c. white basmati rice

1 pt. cream or Half and Half

Simmer carrot, celery, cinnamon, and cloves in the soup stock for 1 hour. Strain. Bring this broth to a boil. Add rice and cook until soft, about 15 minutes. Add spinach, cook for 1 minute. Blend. Add cream and reheat gently.

Strawberry Soup

2 pts. fresh strawberries

1 t. fresh lemon peel

1 c. non-fat yogurt

1/2 c. non-alcoholic champagne

Blend, reserving a strawberry for slicing as a garnish.

Tomato-Mozzarella Salad

2-4 large red-ripe tomatoes in season

1/2 lb. fresh mozzarella cheese

Sprigs of fresh basil

Salt and pepper to taste

Olive oil, high quality

Fresh baguettes

Slice tomatoes and cheese and arrange on a platter. Top with chopped fresh basil, salt, and pepper combined with olive oil. Let flavors blend for 1/2 hour before serving. Serve with fresh baguettes.

SPIRIT-IN-NATURE
ESSENCES INDEX

"The ox is slow, but the earth is patient." —Source unknown

This index affords quick and easy reference for the practitioner and the layperson alike. Here, you will find both positive and negative qualities and conditions listed—in other words, both sides of the essence coin. Coconut, as an example, is listed under willingness *and* unwillingness. The indexed negative qualities are our shortcomings or imperfect attempts at their positive opposite expressions. The positive qualities represent the vibrational message of the essences and we ourselves expressing those qualities, much like the before and after photos that are sometimes used in advertising.

Thus, the index may be used in two ways. You might say, "I'd really like to have more hope," in which case you would refer to that specific category, or "I'm really in a mood today," and check under "Moodiness" and related sections such as "Temperamentalism" and "Unhappiness." After finding the desired subject, you may want to refer to the corresponding essence chapter for complete information on that particular essence.

If you are searching for a quality or condition that is not listed, check under a comparable topic. There are several reasons why a quality may be unlisted in this index: (1) it may be a state such as childhood, for which all the essences apply; (2) as a rule, physical conditions are not listed because, as mentioned earlier, flower essences address psycho-emotional issues and not the physical level directly; or (3) I am still collecting data on those topics.

Abandonment	Grape	Strawberry	
Absent-mindedness	Avocado		
Abundance	Date	Pineapple	
Abuse	Orange	Strawberry	
Acceptance	Apple	Date	
Accident-proneness	Pear		
Accuracy	Avocado		
Achievement	Corn		
Acuity	Avocado		
Adaptability	Fig		
Addiction	Almond	Tomato	
Adjustability	Fig		
Adventure	Spinach		
Advice-seeking	Lettuce		
Advice-giving	Peach		
Affirmation of life	Corn		
Agelessness	Strawberry		
Agitation	Lettuce		
Alertness	Avocado		
Alienation	Grape		
Aloofness	Grape		
Altruism	Peach		
Ambivalence	Strawberry		
Analytical	Spinach		
Anger	Almond	Apple	Lettuce
Anguish	Orange		
Animals, love of	Peach	Spinach	
Annoyance	Date		
Anxiety	Banana	Tomato	
Apathy	Orange		
Apologetic, overly	Strawberry		
Appreciation	Peach	Spinach	
Apprehension	Tomato		

Arrogance	Banana		
Articulateness	Blackberry	Fig	
Attachment, negative	Banana		
Attention	Avocado		
Attitudes, unhealthy	Apple		
Attunement, to others	Date		
Auric disturbances	Pear		
"Autopilot" state	Corn		
Avoidance	Coconut		
Awareness	Avocado	Coconut	
Awareness, environmental	Blackberry		
Awe	Spinach		
Balance	Almond	Apple	Pear
Beauty, love of	Strawberry		
Belief, in self _Joey_	Tomato		
Benevolence	Raspberry		
Bliss	Orange		
Bitterness	Raspberry		
Blame, of others	Grape	Raspberry	
Blocked energy	Corn		
Bluntness	Blackberry		
Body image	Strawberry		
Boredom	Corn		
Boundaries	Fig		
Brashness	Pear		
Break-ups	Strawberry		
Bubbliness	Cherry		
Buoyancy	Spinach		
Burdened	Orange	Spinach	
Calm	Almond	Banana	Lettuce
Care	Peach		
Career problems	Pineapple		
Carefree	Spinach		

Caution	Pear		
Celebration	Tomato		
Centeredness	Pear	Tomato	
Certainty	Lettuce		
Challenges	Avocado	Coconut	
Change	Corn	Tomato	
Character strength	Pineapple		
Cheerfulness	Cherry		
Childbirth	Pear		
Child-likeness	Cherry	Spinach	
Clarity	Avocado	Banana	Blackberry
	Lettuce	Pineapple	
Cleansing	Apple	Blackberry	
Clinginess	Grape		
Closed-minded	Blackberry		
Clouded thinking	Blackberry		
Clumsiness	Strawberry		
Codependence	See Chapter Thirty-two		
Commitment	Coconut	Grape	Strawberry
Common sense	Blackberry		
Communication	Lettuce		
Companionship, unpleasant	Date		
Comparison, self to others	Pineapple	Strawberry	
Compassion	Date	Peach	Raspberry
Competency	Peach		
Complaining nature	Blackberry	Date	
Completion	Coconut		
Composure	Pear		
Compromise, inability to	Fig	Pear	
Compulsion	Fig		
Concentration	Avocado	Lettuce	
Concern	Peach		
Condemnation	Fig		

Confidence *Joeg*	Pineapple		
Conflict	Banana	Orange	Pear
Confrontation	Blackberry		
Confusion	Avocado		
Consideration	Grape	Peach	
Constriction	Peach		
Contentment	Cherry	Date	Pineapple
Contractiveness	Coconut		
Contrariness	Cherry		
Control, lack of	Almond	Cherry	
Courage	Tomato		
Courteousness	Grape	Strawberry	
Conviction, lack of	Tomato		
Cowardice	Tomato		
Creativity	Corn	Lettuce	
Crisis	Pear		
Criticism	Date	Fig	Grape
Crowds	Tomato		
Cruelty	Blackberry	Grape	Raspberry
Curiosity	Spinach		
Cynicism	Blackberry		
Dark thoughts	Blackberry		
Dauntlessness	Tomato		
Daydreaming	Avocado		
Death, grieving	Grape		
Deception	Blackberry		
Decisiveness	Lettuce	Strawberry	
Defeatism	Coconut	Tomato	
Defensiveness	Banana	Tomato	
Demand	Grape		
Denial	Blackberry		
Dependability	Strawberry		
Depression	Orange	Peach	

Emergency	Pear		
Emotions	Apple	Grape	Lettuce
	Orange	Raspberry	
Empathy	Raspberry		
Empowerment	Tomato		
Emptiness	Grape		
Endurance	Coconut	Corn	Orange
Energy	Corn		
Enjoyment	Spinach		
Enthusiasm	Corn	Orange	Spinach
Environmental awareness	Blackberry		
Envy	Grape		
Escapism	Coconut		
Evasiveness	Blackberry		
Even-mindedness	Cherry		
Excess	Almond		
Excuses, making	Coconut		
Exhaustion	Corn		
Expansion	Coconut	Grape	
Expectations, unrealistic	Grape	Fig	
Exploitation	Peach		
Exploration	Spinach		
Exuberance	Spinach		
Failure	Lettuce	Tomato	
Fanaticism	Fig		
Fault-finding	Blackberry	Cherry	
Fear	Apple	Spinach	Tomato
Fearlessness	Apple	Tomato	
Fear of aging	Strawberry		
Flexibility	Fig		
Fluidity	Fig	Pear	
Focus	Avocado	Blackberry	
Forgetfulness	Avocado		

Forgiveness	Raspberry		
Frailty	Tomato		
Freedom	Spinach		
Friction	Pear		
Friendliness	Spinach		
Friendship	Grape		
Frigidity	Grape		
Frugality	Blackberry		
Frustration	Almond	Blackberry	
Garrulousness	Peach		
Generosity	Peach	Raspberry	
Gentleness	Banana	Blackberry	Peach
Gloom	Cherry		
Goodness	Blackberry		
Gossip	Blackberry		
Gracefulness	Strawberry		
Greatness	Banana		
Greed	Grape	Peach	
Grief	Grape	Orange	Pear
Groundedness	Strawberry		
Grudges	Raspberry		
Grumpiness	Cherry		
Guidance	Fig		
Guilt	Peach	Strawberry	
Guilelessness	Spinach		
Habit-bound	Almond		
Happiness	Apple	Cherry	
Harmony	Pear		
Hastiness	Pear		
Healthfulness	Apple		
Heart	Cherry	Grape	Raspberry
Heaviness	Cherry	Orange	
Helpfulness	Peach	Raspberry	

Hesitation	Tomato		
Homesickness	Avocado		
Honesty	Pineapple	Spinach	
Honor	Blackberry	Coconut	
Hope	Apple	Cherry	Orange
	Tomato		
Hopelessness	Orange		
Humanitarianism	Pear		
Humility	Banana		
Humor	Blackberry	Fig	Spinach
Hurt feelings	Raspberry		
Hypochondria	Apple	Fig	
Identity, sense of	Pineapple		
Illness, fear of	Apple	Tomato	
Immoderation	Almond		
Imposition	Pineapple		
Impotence	Grape		
Impurity	Apple	Blackberry	
Inadaptability	Fig		
Inadequacy	Peach	Strawberry	
Inattention	Avocado		
Incisiveness	Blackberry		
Inconsideration	Grape	Peach	
Indecisiveness	Apple	Lettuce	Strawberry
Inferiority complex	Pineapple		
Inhibitions	Fig	Tomato	
Inhospitable	Date		
Initiative	Corn		
Innocence	Blackberry	Spinach	
Innovation	Corn		
Insecurity	Strawberry		
Insensitivity	Peach	Raspberry	
Insight	Blackberry		

Inspiration	Blackberry	Cherry	Grape
Instability	Tomato		
Insults	Blackberry		
Integration	Apple	Orange	
Integrity	Strawberry		
Intellectual	Spinach		
Interest	Peach	Spinach	
Interest in life	Orange		
Interiorization	Almond		
Intimacy	Grape		
Intolerance	Date		
Introspection	Blackberry		
Intuition	Fig		
Invincibility	Tomato		
Inwardness	Almond		
Irascibility	Date		
Irresolution	Orange		
Irresponsibility	Strawberry		
Irritability	Date		
Jealousy	Apple	Grape	
Joy	Corn	Orange	Peach
	Spinach		
Judged, feeling	Fig	Pineapple	
Judgment	Banana	Blackberry	Date
	Fig		
Kindheartedness	Raspberry		
Kindness	Blackberry	Peach	Raspberry
Lackluster attitude	Corn		
Lashing out	Raspberry		
Laughter	Cherry		
Laziness	Corn		
Lessons	Avocado		
Lethargy	Corn		

Letting go	Raspberry		
Lightheartedness	Cherry		
Lightness	Cherry	Orange	
Limitations	Fig	Pineapple	
Listening	Banana	Date	Peach
	Raspberry		
Loneliness	Date	Grape	Peach
Lost, feeling	Strawberry		
Loudness	Pineapple		
Love	Grape	Peach	Pear
	Raspberry		
Love of beauty	Strawberry		
Lust	Grape		
Magnetism	Apple	Date	Grape
Manipulation	Peach		
Martyrdom	Fig	Peach	
Maturity	Blackberry	Peach	Strawberry
Meanness	Blackberry	Raspberry	
Meddlesome	Peach		
Melancholia	Orange		
Memory	Avocado		
Menopause	See Chapter Thirty-two		
Mindfulness	Avocado		
Mischievousness	Spinach		
Mistakes	Avocado		
Moderation	Almond		
Modesty	Banana		
Money issues	Pineapple		
Moodiness	Cherry		
Morality	Blackberry		
Narrowness	Date	Peach	
Nastiness	Raspberry		
Nature, sharing	Spinach		

Neediness	Grape	Peach	
Negative emotions	Grape		
Negativity	Banana	Blackberry	Cherry
	Orange		
Nervousness	Almond	Banana	Lettuce
	Pear		
Nightmares	Tomato		
Non-acceptance	Date		
Non-commitment	Avocado	Coconut	Grape
Non-possessiveness	Grape		
Non-reactiveness	Banana		
Nurturance	Grape	Peach	
Obedience, expecting	Grape		
Objectivity	Banana		
Obnoxiousness	Pineapple		
Observance, quality of	Banana		
Obsessiveness	Fig		
Obstinacy	Banana		
Open-mindedness	Date	Fig	
Openness	Avocado	Tomato	
Opinionated	Banana		
Optimism	Blackberry	Cherry	
Organization	Avocado		
Orneriness	Cherry		
"Out of sorts"	Pear		
Outrageousness	Blackberry	Pineapple	
Outspokenness	Pineapple		
Overbearing	Grape	Pineapple	
Overburden	Spinach		
Over-concern	Apple		
Over-conscientiousness	Strawberry		
Over-extending	Fig		
Overindulgence	Almond		

Overly-serious	Fig	Spinach	
Over-reactiveness	Raspberry		
Oversensitivity	Strawberry		
Overwhelm	Avocado	Spinach	
Nature, attunement with	Spinach		
Pain	Orange		
Paranoia	Spinach		
Past issues	Avocado		
Patience	Coconut	Grape	Lettuce
Peace	Banana	Grape	Pear
Peacemaker	Pear		
Peace of mind	Pear		
Perfectionism	Fig		
Perseverance	Coconut	Orange	
Perspective, loss of	Banana		
Pessimism	Blackberry	Cherry	
Pioneering spirit	Corn		
Playfulness	Spinach		
Pliancy	Fig		
Playfulness	Spinach		
Poise	Strawberry		
Positivity	Cherry		
Possessiveness	Grape		
Potential	Coconut		
Poverty consciousness	Pineapple		
Power	Pineapple		
Practicality	Strawberry		
Prejudice	Date	Fig	
Present, living fully in	Avocado	Corn	Pear
Pride	Banana	Pineapple	Strawberry
Problem-oriented	Coconut		
Procrastination	Coconut	Corn	
Projects	Avocado		

Repression	Lettuce		
Resentment	Raspberry		
Resignation	Orange		
Resilience	Orange		
Respect	Grape	Spinach	Strawberry
Responsibility	Date	Raspberry	Strawberry
Responsiveness	Corn		
Restlessness	Almond	Lettuce	
Reverence	Orange		
Rhythm, sense of	Pear		
Rigidity	Fig		
Rudeness	Peach		
Sadness	Cherry		
Sarcasm	Blackberry		
Satisfaction	Spinach		
Scatteredness	Lettuce		
Security	Peach		
Self-acceptance	Fig		
Self-assuredness	Pineapple		
Self-blame	Blackberry	Strawberry	
Self-care	Apple		
Self-control	Almond		
Self-critical	Fig		
Self-denial	Fig		
Self-dominating	Fig		
Self-honesty	Blackberry	Tomato	
Self-involvement	Peach		
Selfishness	Peach		
Selflessness	Peach		
Self-liberation	Fig		
Self-limitation	Fig		
Self-nurturance	Date		
Self-pity	Cherry	Orange	

Straightforwardness	Blackberry		
Strength	Apple	Banana	Coconut
	Date	Pear	Tomato
Stress	Almond	Spinach	Tomato
Strictness	Fig		
Struggle	Orange		
Substance abuse	Almond	Tomato	
"Stuck," feeling	Corn		
Success	Lettuce	Tomato	
Suffering	Orange		
Supportiveness	Peach		
Suppression	Fig		
Surrender	Banana		
Sweetness	Date		
Sweets, craving	Date		
Sympathy	Raspberry		
Synchronicity	Almond		
Taciturn	Banana		
Tactlessness	Blackberry	Pineapple	
Tastes, refined	Strawberry		
Teasing	Grape		
Temperamentalism	Cherry		
Temperance	Almond		
Tenderness	Date		
Tension	Fig	Pear	Spinach
Terror	Tomato		
Thoughts, quality of	Apple		
Thoughtlessness	Peach		
Tolerance	Fig	Lettuce	
Touchiness	Raspberry		
Trauma	Pear		
Transcendence	Grape	Orange	
Travel	Tomato		

Vitality	Corn	Orange	
Vulnerability	Apple	Grape	Pear
Weakness	Tomato		
Weariness	Corn		
Welcoming	Date		
Well-being	Almond	Apple	
Wholeness	Apple		
Wholesomeness	Apple		
Willingness	Avocado	Coconut	Corn
	Pear		
Will power	Corn	Tomato	
Wisdom	Date	Fig	Pineapple
	Raspberry		
Withdrawal	Tomato		
Withdrawn nature	Lettuce		
Wonderment	Spinach		
"Workaholic"	Almond		
Worry	Apple	Spinach	
Woundedness	Raspberry		
Zeal	Corn		

ENDNOTES

1   Tompkins, Peter and Christopher Bird, *The Secret Life of Plants*, Harper & Row, New York, NY, 1973, p. 97.

2   Ibid., p. 103.

3   Clark, Glenn, *The Man Who Talks With the Flowers*, Macalester Park Publishing Co., Saint Paul, MN, 1939, pp. 22-23.

4   Ibid., p. 40.

5   Frawley, David and Dr. Vasant Lad, *The Yoga of Herbs*, Lotus Press, Santa Fe, NM, 1986, p. 6.

6   Clark, p. 45.

7   Yogananda, Paramhansa, *Autobiography of a Yogi*, The Philosophical Library, Inc., New York, NY 1946, reprint by Crystal Clarity Publishers, Nevada City, CA, 1994, p. 348.

8   Ibid., p. 377.

9   Anderson, John E., "What Makes Olympic Champions?" *Reader's Digest*, February, 1994.

10   Yogananda, p. 438.

11   Ma, Ananda Moi, *Matri Darshan*, Mangalam Verlag S. Schang, Germany, 1983.

12   Yogananda, p. 147.

13   Hotchner, A. H., *Sophia: Living And Loving*, William Morrow and Company, Inc., New York, NY, 1979, p. 251.

14   Hendrix, Harville, *Keeping the Love You Find*, Simon & Schuster Inc., New York, NY, 1992, p. 11.

15   Stewart-Wallace, Sir John and Swami Ghanananda, *Women Saints East & West*, Vedanta Press, Hollywood, CA, 1955, p. 65.

BIBLIOGRAPHY

Academic American Encyclopedia, Grolier, Inc. Danbury, CT, 1995.

Anderson, John E., "What Makes Olympic Champions?," *Reader's Digest,* February, 1994.

Ashe, Arthur, and Arnold Rampersad, *Days Of Grace,* Alfred A. Knopf, New York, NY, 1993.

Askew, Judith S., *Menopause News,* "Stunning Statistics," July/August 1992, San Francisco, CA.

Barbach, Lonnie, *The Pause,* Penguin Books, New York, NY, 1993.

Beatie, Melody, *Codependent No More,* Harper & Row, San Francisco, CA, 1987.

Ball, Ann, *Modern Saints: Their Lives and Faces,* Tan Books and Publishers, Inc., Rockford, IL, 1983.

Benet, William Rose, *The Reader's Encyclopedia,* Thomas Y Corwell Company, New York, NY, 1965.

Bio-Academic American Encyclopedia, Grolier, Inc , Danbury, CT, 1995.

Burbank, Luther, *Plant Breeding: Volume I,* P. F. Collier & Son Company, New York, NY, 1921.

Canfield, Jack, and Mark Victor Hansen, *Chicken Soup For The Soul,* Health Communications, Inc., Deerfield Beach, FL, 1993.

Castro, Miranda, *The Complete Homeopathy Handbook,* St. Martin's Press, New York, NY, 1991.

Clark, Glenn, *The Man Who Talks With The Flowers*, Macalester Park Publishing Co., Saint Paul, MN, 1993.

Coffee, Timothy, *The History and Folklore of North American Wildflowers*, Facts on File, Inc., New York, NY, 1993.

Frawley, David and Dr. Vasant Lad, *The Yoga of Herbs*, Lotus Press, Santa Fe, NM, 1986.

Hawking, Stephen W., *A Brief History Of Time*, Bantam Books, New York, NY, 1988.

Heinerman, John, *Heinerman's Encyclopedia of Fruits, Vegetables and Herbs*, Parker Publishing Co., West Nyack, NY, 1988.

Hotchner, A. H., *Sophia: Living And Loving*, William Morrow and Company, Inc., New York, NY, 1979.

Hendrix, Harville, *Keeping the Love You Find*, Simon & Schuster Inc., New York, NY, 1992.

Jensen, Dr. Bernard, *Foods That Heal*, Avery Publishing Group, Inc., Garden City Park, NY, 1988.

Kadans, Joseph M., *Encyclopedia Of Fruits, Vegetables, Nuts And Seeds For Healthful Living*, Parker Publishing Co., New York, NY, 1973.

Ma, Ananda Moi, *Matri Darshan*, Mangalam Verlag S. Schang, Germany, 1983.

Mair, Nancy and Bhakti Rinzler, *Simply Vegetarian*, Dawn Publications, Nevada City, CA, 1985.

Masefield, G. B., M. Wallis and S. G. Harrison, *The Oxford Book of Food Plants*, Oxford University Press, London, 1969.

Miller, Carey D., Katherine Bazore, and Mary Bartow, *Fruits of Hawaii*, University of Hawaii, Honolulu, HI, 1955.

Milne, A. A., *The World of Pooh*, Methuen Children's Books, London, England, 1958.

Mohan-Mala: A Gandhian Rosary, Navajivan Publishing House, Ahmedabad, India, 1949.

Mukerji, Bithika, *From the Life of Sri Anandamayi Ma*, Shreeshree Ananda Mayee Charitable Society, Calcutta, India, 1980.

Norwood, Robin, *Women Who Love Too Much*, Pocket Books, New York, NY, 1985.

Rodale, J. I., *Encyclopedia of Organic Gardening*, Rodale Books, Inc., Emmaus, PA, 1969.

Ruffin, C. Bernard, *Padre Pio: The True Story*, Our Sunday Visitor, Inc., Huntington, IN, 1982.

Shoesteck, Robert, *Flowers And Plants*, The New York Times Book Co., New York, NY, 1974.

Smith, Penelope, *Animal Talk*, Pegasus Publications, Point Reyes Station, CA 1989.

Stewart-Wallace, John and Swami Ghanananda, *Women Saints East & West*, Vedanta Press, Hollywood, CA, 1955.

Swenson, Allan A., *Landscape You Can Eat*, David McKay Company, Inc., New York, NY, 1977.

Tompkins, Peter, and Christopher Bird, *The Secret Life of Plants*, Harper & Row Publishers, New York, NY, 1973.

Travers, P. L., *Mary Poppins*, Harcourt Brace, New York, NY, 1934.

Walters, J. Donald, *Your Sun Sign as a Spiritual Guide*, Crystal Clarity Publishers, Nevada City, CA, 1983.

On Wings Of Joy, Crystal Clarity Publishers, 1987.

Wynne, Peter, *Apples*, Hawthorn Books, Inc., New York, 1975.

Yogananda, Paramhansa, *Autobiography of a Yogi*, The Philosophical Library, Inc., New York, NY, 1946, reprint by Crystal Clarity Publishers, Nevada City, CA, 1994.

The Rubaiyat Of Omar Khayyam, Explained, Paramhansa Yogananda, J. Donald Walters, ed., Crystal Clarity Publishers, Nevada City, CA, 1994.

PRODUCTS AND PROGRAMS

PRODUCTS

Individual Stock Concentrate Bottles in 1/2 oz. (15 ml.) and 1 oz. (30 ml.) sizes: In cobalt blue glass bottles with full-color designer labels on a golden water-color background, high quality glass pipettes, and tamper-proof shrink bands. Spirit-in-Nature Essences are prepared from the purest blossoms in their peak of bloom. To ensure their full shelf life, store them upright and out of heat and humidity.

Practitioner Kit: Complete kit of 20 1/2 oz. (15 ml.) Stock Concentrate Bottled in a purple cardboard box with dividers, outer label and inside grid, 4"x 4"x 6," providing a handy package for travel and storage.

Professional Set: Full set of 20 1 oz. (30 ml.) Stock Bottles in 2 attractive blue cardboard 13"x 4"x 1-5/8" boxes, ideal for home or professional use.

Flower Essences for Animals: Remedies for Helping The Pets You Love, by Lila Devi, 272 pages, softcover. This book presents a bird's eye view into the animal kingdom. It offers a treasury of practical tools for enhancing the quality of the lives of your beloved animal companions. Addressing specific conditions and behaviors, this book provides simple solutions for administering the best possible pet care in both daily life and emergency situations.

Bradley Banana and the Jolly Good Pirate is the first of 20 hardcover children's picture books, each personifying a flower essence's uplifting quality in a thrilling adventure.

Affirmation Deck: This deck of 20 cards, plus two additional instruction cards, in a handsomely designed jeweled matte laminate gift box (4"x 6"x 1-1/4") includes brilliant blossom and fruit photos with rhythmical affirmations. Spirit-in-Nature Essences act much like "bottled affirmations," while affirmations might be called "verbal essences." Since both help to awaken the positive qualities within our nature, using them interactively will increase their effectiveness.

Mini-poster: A full-color, 8"x10" on glossy cardstock, suitable for framing. This stunning reference chart reflects a compilation of decades of collected flower photos, updated essence definitions, and vivid color and design. It features the Essence Spectrum Chart along with a text explanation. The screened background of lush fruits serves as a visual reminder of "the flower/food connection." Beautifully rendered by graphic designer Chitra Sudhakaran, this at-a-glance chart brings Spirit-in-Nature Essences to life, enlivening their subtle energies.

Pet Mini-Poster: As above with our regular mini-poster, our pets version in antique gold, offers adapted information on a screened background of pets and animals. This frame-worthy rendition honors our animal friends and their flower essence needs.

Pear Spray (for people and pets): 1 oz. (30 ml.) and **Pear, Grape,** and **Tomato Spary** (15 ml.) Stock Bottles are "liquid peace, love, and courage," respectively. Keep them handy at all times!

CD-ROM Tour: Take a 59-slide tour of Spirit-in-Nature Essences on your computer. This presentation includes 20 blossom/essence slides, 20 FAQ pages and other helpful information, with a rich display of photos and graphics. Use it for your personal study, for reference, or for teaching.

DVD Video Series of 21 short video clips, one per essence and an introductory video. Includes stunning graphics, photos, affirmations, and background music, narrated by founder Lila Devi.

"Essence Songs": a lively CD featuring compositions by J. Donald Walters and sung by Mr. Walters and the Ananda World Brotherhood Choir. Each of these songs musically and lyrically conveys the message of its corresponding essence.

Dosage Bottle Labels: Created by graphic artist Sara Cryer, these designer labels will highlight your formulas. The gold watercolor background provides an artistic and professional label for your bottles, 1-oz. or larger. Measuring 2"h x 3-3/4"w, they match the design of our regular Stock Concentrate labels, with blank lines to write a name, formula, date, and directions.

Retail, wholesale, and distributor information is available on request.

PROGRAMS

Comprehensive Home Study Course with Certification: Our course includes three levels, each with certification. This cumulative course offers an internationally acclaimed study of the art of flower essences featuring Spirit-in-Nature Essences and provides excellent training for laypeople and practitioners. Enroll in one, two, or three levels.

Pets and Animals Home Study Course with Certification: This course includes two levels, each with certification, with training in the application of Spirit-in-Nature Essences for natural pet care. Animal lovers worldwide report that this course helps them to improve the lives of the pets they love through the gentle yet powerful medium of flower essences. Enroll in one or both levels.

Please visit our website (updated regularly) for information on upcoming seminars, workshops, and other events. To arrange programs in your area, please contact us at:

Spirit-in-Nature Essences
14618 Tyler Foote Road
Nevada City, CA 95959 USA
Tel 530.478.7655
Fax .530.478.7652
Toll free ordering: 800.347.3639
www.Spirit-in-Nature.com
info@Spirit-in-Nature.com